Drugs and information control

Contributions in Legal Studies
Series Editor: *Paul L. Murphy*

Popular Influence Upon Public Policy: Petitioning in Eighteenth-Century Virginia
Raymond C. Bailey

Fathers to Daughters: The Legal Foundations of Female Emancipation
Peggy A. Rabkin

In Honor of Justice Douglas: A Symposium on Individual Freedom and the Government
Robert H. Keller, Jr., editor

A Constitutional History of Habeas Corpus
William F. Duker

The American Codification Movement: A Study of Antebellum Legal Reform
Charles M. Cook

Crime and Punishment in Revolutionary Paris
Antoinette Wills

American Legal Culture, 1908-1940
John W. Johnson

Governmental Secrecy and the Founding Fathers: A Study in Constitutional Controls
Daniel N. Hoffman

Torture and English Law: An Administrative and Legal History from the Plantagenets to the Stuarts
James Heath

Essays on New York Colonial Legal History
Herbert S. Johnson

The Origins of the American Business Corporation, 1784-1855: Broadening the Concept of Public Service During Industrialization
Ronald E. Seavoy

Prologue to Nuremberg: The Politics and Diplomacy of Punishing War Criminals of the First World War
James F. Willis

The Network of Control: State Supreme Courts and State Security Statutes, 1920-1970
Carol E. Jenson

Drugs and information control

THE ROLE OF MEN AND MANIPULATION IN THE CONTROL OF DRUG TRAFFICKING

JERALD W. CLOYD

CONTRIBUTIONS IN LEGAL STUDIES, NUMBER 23

Greenwood Press
WESTPORT, CONNECTICUT • LONDON, ENGLAND

Copyright Acknowledgment

Grateful acknowledgment is given to the journal *Social Problems* and to The Society for the Study of Social Problems for permission to use edited excerpts from "Prosecution's Power, Procedural Rights, and Pleading Guilty: The Problems of Coercion in Plea Bargaining Drug Cases," by Jerald Cloyd, which appeared in *Social Problems,* vol. 26, no. 4 (April 1979): 452-66.

Library of Congress Cataloging in Publication Data

Cloyd, Jerald W.
    Drugs and information control.

    (Contributions in legal studies, ISSN 0147-1074;
no. 23)
    Bibliography: p.
    Includes index.
    1. Drug abuse—United States. 2. Narcotic laws—
United States. 3. Narcotics, Control of—United States.
I. Title. II. Series.
HV5825.C58   363.4'5'0973   81-6675
ISBN 0-313-22178-2 (lib. bdg.)   AACR2

Library of Congress Catalog Card Number: 81-6675
ISBN: 0-313-22178-2
ISSN: 0147-1074

First published in 1982

Greenwood Press
A division of Congressional Information Service, Inc.
88 Post Road West, Westport, Connecticut 06881

Printed in the United States of America

10 9 8 7 6 5 4 3 2 1

To Joe and Jack

CONTENTS

TABLES

PREFACE

The increased interest in drugs since 1966 has given rise to a number of new and important studies concerning the origin, causes, and present status of drug use in the United States. Many of these studies have been scholarly and have been based extensively on primary sources, including historical documents concerning the rise of drug use, antidrug legislation at the turn of the century, and current documents outlining present drug use and control policies. Although these studies often espouse different theoretical perspectives, their focusing on a multiplicity of facts in order to support these perspectives makes for somewhat laborious reading, especially for the lay audience.

This book is written for both the lay audience and scholars and attempts to focus on the essential aspects of the drug problem: cultural context, laws prohibiting drug use, and present control procedures. Footnotes have been used to guide readers to those primary sources on which this book is based, but I have made no attempt to replicate the detail of these original studies. Rather this book attempts to provide an overview of the history of the major drugs used in the United States today (opiates, cocaine, and marijuana) as well as contemporary drug control policies. Much of the material concerning contemporary drug control policies was derived from extensive interviews and personal observation of law enforcement personnel. Of special concern throughout this work is the role of information in the interpretation, expansion, and control of the drug experience.

I am indebted to a number of people for crucial insights into both the existential-conflict paradigm and the substantive importance of information control in developing power. My mentors at the University of California at San Diego were very helpful in pointing out the theoretical importance of the existential perspective, as well as the centrality of social conflict in understanding the place of intoxicants in our society. Joseph Gusfield and Jack Douglas at the University of California at San Diego, John Johnson at Arizona State University, and Carol A. B. Warren at the University of Southern California all have made this theoretical paradigm significant and, in their own ways, made this book possible. I am most indebted to Barbara Minor, who showed me that for information control to be legitimate and, hopefully, of a lasting quality, it must be based on a fundamental respect for social decency.

Drugs and information control

INTRODUCTION
THE DRUG ISSUE: THEORETICAL PERSPECTIVES CONCERNING THE SIGNIFICANCE OF INFORMATION CONTROL

The literature on drugs has increased enormously since 1966. With the apparent rise of drug use among the middle class, social scientists have given increased attention to this topic. From a sociological perspective, a central issue concerns the inherently problematic nature of both drug use and the legal processes designated for its control. As Douglas remarked in his study of drug use during the early 1970s, "There is always some unpredictability in the effects of drugs and always some unpredictability in the drug problem."[1] At the individual level, the effects of drugs on a particular user may range from states of euphoric bliss to anxiety and depression. The problematic aspects of the drug issue are also reflected within the larger social order, with conflicting views surrounding the moral value of drug use. Although most of Western history has reflected little overt social concern with drug use, the last hundred years has witnessed a considerable increase in social and legal attention to this activity. The reasons for this increased social concern, as well as the legitimacy of the legal sanctions created for its control, have been the object of much public and scholarly dialogue, as well as diatribe.

My purpose in this study is to focus on a central feature of all aspects of the drug issue—the role of information control. Specifically, the focus will be on the role of information control within the social context in which drugs are used, the societal context in which antidrug laws are created, and the legal context in which law enforcement agencies attempt to enforce these drug laws. By information control I mean the conscious collection, formation, and distribution of information within each of these social contexts. The labelling theorists have been the most prolific and influential in delineating this topic during the last several decades. They suggest that the drug problem is socially created when an individual or group consciously defines (labels) drug use as negative. Because they acknowledge the problematic features of drug use and traffic, as well as the importance of information control in the social interpretation of this issue, this perspective is a natural theoretical point of departure.

LABELLING THEORY: THE ROLE OF INFORMATION IN THE CREATION OF DEVIANCE

Given the varied effects that drugs can have on individual users, the way in which this information is used, or the way an individual interprets their experiences is crucial to the creation of a relatively stable understanding of these effects. Becker stated in his classic work in this area that

the effects of the drug, when first perceived, may be physically unpleasant or at least ambiguous ... the novice's naive interpretation of what is happening to him may further confuse and frighten him, particularly if he decides, as many do, that he is going insane.... [However], the more experienced user ... teaches him to regard those ambiguous experiences formerly defined as unpleasant as enjoyable.... In short, what was once frightening and distasteful becomes, after a taste for it is built up, pleasant, desired, and sought after.[2]

Through interaction between the user and his peers, a social meaning is constructed and the experience is labelled "pleasant."

Becker has also acknowledged the importance of information control in the structuring of antidrug legislation by those who do not share the drug users' "pleasant" interpretation of its effects. Just as individual users are guided toward a particular interpretation of their experience by significant individuals, so the larger legal definition of drug use becomes the product of information control by influential individuals within the political realm. What Becker describes as the "moral entrepreneur" is the fundamental force behind the antidrug legislative movement. This individual is zealously concerned with the negative aspects of drug use and fanatically generates and coordinates a legislative effort to control its misuse. Central to this effort is the control of information at conferences, through the mass media, and within congressional hearings. This manipulation of information, in turn, creates an emotional antidrug environment within key sectors of the legislative structure, as well as the public at large. Hence, the social momentum necessary for passage of these acts, like the individual user's interpretation of the actual drug experience, can be traced back to an individual who is acting within a specific social context.

Although Becker's work has been a major contribution to a theoretical perspective on the drug problem, more recent work in this area indicates that it is too simplistic. Becker's view incorporates an assumption that sees a linear causal nexus between the activities of the moral entrepreneur and the creation of the label that defines drug use as deviant. Douglas critiques this assumption from an existential point of view. As an existentialist he is suspicious of a simple causal explanation of social behavior and emphasizes a more problematic and multidimentional approach. Douglas states that "labelling theorists have recognized the problematic nature of the categories of morality, but they took the imputation process themselves as nonproblematic."[3] Douglas argues that many of the traditional labelling theorists—Becker, Lindesmith, Lemert, and Tannenbaum—have tended to underplay the importance of several other factors in this labelling process. That is, they have not entertained the possibility of a more complex causal nexus at work in generating a legal statement on the drug issue. Specifically, these theorists tend to assume that structural influences, such as economic trends or class and racial tensions, are not a crucial force behind this process. Rather, the individual moral entrepreneur is responsible for arousing the latent class antagonisms that might fuel his antidrug crusade, but the individual is not viewed as the pawn of these structural dynamics. Further, the labelling perspective assumes that these antidrug laws have a significant degree of emotional charge but do not adequately address the form, degree, or manner in which this aspect of the label is created. Finally, traditional labelling theorists have not expanded beyond the unilinear notion of the moral entrepreneur's control of information that directly sparks public emotions against drug use and, ultimately, fosters the antidrug legislation.

Although the labelling theorists remain weak on these three points, more contemporary theorists have attempted to move beyond at least the last objection. Specifically, Albert Hess[4] has indicated that a close examination of the information process that generated the first anti-drug legislation in 1914 reveals the existence of a more complex information system than the unilinear modes envisioned by the traditional labelling theorists. He argues that around the turn of the century, an informational feedback loop existed between those who generated the laws (moral entrepreneurs) and those who became the victims. This concept of a feedback loop emphasizes a circular flow of information from those who originally had drug experiences to those who labelled these experiences as deviant, which in turn created a negative legal sanction on the drug user. He argues further that these legal sanctions are not due to the zealous momentum of a single individual, or possibly a particular political lobby, but rather arise more slowly out of the inherently unpredictable nature of the drug experience itself. The effects of drugs always produce numerous conflicting interpretations. Some experiences will be interpreted positively because of the particular social context in which they arise, as Becker described, others will be interpreted as negative, and these too will gain circulation. Ultimately, according to Hess, this negative information set became dominant and set up a feedback loop between those who interpreted drug use in a positive light and those, especially nondrug users, who interpreted its use as essentially negative. The political figures (moral entrepreneurs) rode the negative definition through the legislature and gained the passage of the desired legal sanctions, an action that further alienated the users from the larger society and created a separate and isolated class of deviants.

This more innovative approach is important, but Hess's perspective is constrained by a number of limitations inherent in the labelling perspective. Although he does address the problematic nature of the drug issue and the role of information in the structuring of a workable social definition of it, he does not explain the factors that cause one definition to dominate over competing ones. As Becker's work indicates, there can be both a positive and/or negative interpretation of the drug experience, with the positive definition having at least a partial following. Hess alludes to variables beyond the information structure, but because he is primarily concerned with the process of information flow, he does not develop his analysis. Douglas, Warren, and Johnson, however, focus on this problem when they point out that "perhaps the most fundamental existential problem with labelling theory is its abstracting of [social definitions or labels] from the context of uses and situations [surrounding] the actors on the actual occasions of their use."[5]

Although some recent labelling theorists have attempted to grapple with the problem of complex information feedback systems, the other shortcomings remain inherent within the labelling perspective. A comprehensive theoretical paradigm is needed to incorporate the structural elements of the social order, the specific ways in which these elements organize the members' emotions, and the resulting information feedback loops. Such a paradigm will move easily between microsocial and macrosocial levels.

EXISTENTIAL-CONFLICT THEORY: AN ALTERNATIVE APPROACH TO THE DRUG ISSUE

The situational contexts in which the definitions (labels and laws) are generated and commonly used constitute the rudimentary parts of the larger class or structural dynamics of the social order. By abstracting the labelling process from these situational contexts, the labelling theorists preclude the possibility of investigating the effects that the larger social and historical trends may have on the construction of these laws. The recent theoretical development of the new existential-conflict perspective has set the groundwork for a perspective that goes beyond this limitation. This view, like labelling theory, focuses on the concrete lived experience, or existential reality, of those being studied, but it also moves easily into the more general theoretical concepts that address historical and structural trends. This view has been represented in the empirical studies of Douglas, Cicourel, Johnson, Warren, and others,[6] but one of the most thorough statements at the strictly theoretical level has come from Randall Collins. Collins is aware that the existential foundations of society are "real people in real places, or the writing and artifacts that they have made."[7] However, he is also aware of the need for "concepts that summarize long-term and large-scale networks of interaction, the macro level of analysis."[8] Rather than abstracting the labelling process from the larger structural context, he has synthesized and integrated a number of traditional perspectives (those of Weber, Marx, Michels, and Goffman, among others) into a holistic theoretical paradigm. When he uses terms such as "class," "stratification," "mass media," and "the state," he always refers to actual networks of individuals interacting on a day-to-day basis. Society is always an "aggregate of individuals, groups, and organizations [which act] on the basis of mutual accommodation of their interests—ideal and material—and of the domination of some individuals over others."[9] From these concepts, Collins has developed a perspective that moves easily between the existential description of the activities of actual individuals and the long-term and large-scale networks that have been the dominant focus of traditional sociological thought.

Not only does the existential-conflict perspective provide theoretical flexibility between the microlevel and macrolevel, but it also addresses a number of issues that explain the domination of one feedback loop over other competing loops. Specifically, this perspective, like that of the labelling theorists, sees the amount of emotion infused in a given feedback loop as a key element in the power of that social definition. However, labelling theorists traditionally have made an unwarranted assumption concerning the interface between the cognitive and emotional elements of the labelling process. They have not accurately outlined the relationship between the cognitions or mutual categories of "right" or "wrong" behavior and the human emotions of pleasure, fear, and confusion, which influence the placing of these ideas on specific behavior. Rather than seeing this interface as problematic, as the existential-conflict theorists suggest, labelling theorists have assumed that cognitive processes would dominate and constrain the emotional elements. For example, Becker's description of individual drug users and the activities of moral entrepreneurs suggests that once a label has been placed over the ambivalent feelings inherent in each situation, the social context becomes stabilized. The individual user regards the drug experience as pleasant, and the social order becomes satisfied with the moral entrepreneur's definition of drug abuse. From the labelling perspective, emotions are seen as initially ambivalent but are ultimately dominated and stabilized by individual or social cognitive constructions.

Labelling theorists also assume that ultimately the emotional content of a label can be traced to feelings directly tied to the behavior in question. That is, they assume that the social emotions supporting antidrug legislation arise strictly from public sentiment surrounding this issue, without entertaining the possibility that unrelated issues can be fused with the drug issue and give this legislation added momentum. Hence, from the labelling perspective, antidrug laws can be understood as a direct emotional response to drug abuse, and this emotional charge is safely contained within the labelling process itself. The interface between antidrug feelings and the legislative process is direct, unilinear, and nonproblematic.

The existential-conflict theorists, on the other hand, do not make these assumptions. Instead they assume that the interface between social emotions and the rise of cognitive labels can take numerous forms, with the exact form an empirical rather than a theoretically binding question. Much of what passes for objective cognitive knowledge, these theorists hold, is actually the result of deeper emotional currents. As Collins suggests, "Human beings are animals and human social ties are fundamentally based on automatically aroused emotional responses."[10] This bedrock of the existential position is more colorfully stated by Douglas, who suggests that "to present the whole picture of man we must begin at the beginning, the foundations and ends of all else—feelings. We begin with what Merleau Ponti called 'brute being.'"[11] The "brute being" is always pulling at the bit of the mental processes that attempts to control, constrain, or contour the problematic and open-ended nature of human existence. "Feelings lie behind, are the foundation of, the goal of all thought."[12] Hence, the existentialists, unlike the labelling theorists, argue that the exact relationship between feelings and the process through which this information is translated into cognitive labels (social definitions or laws) has to be teased out of the actual empirical networks in which it is produced. The probability of a complex structural interplay is not a simple unilinear relationship between social feelings and their cognitive products and is always present.

At this point the existential-conflict perspective is compatible with the more traditional structural-conflict theorists. Rather than limiting the analysis to the microlevel of individuals, the existential-conflict perspective readily addresses the larger class and structural tensions that historically infuse powerful, if unrelated, emotions into the drug issue. Specifically, class tensions due to an economic downturn and/or racial hostilities due to migration patterns may be essentially unrelated to the drug issue but can become emotionally fused with that issue and give it momentum. The mercurial nature of emotions provides the resource for one social definition to dominate over its competitors. The successful definition of social reality is the product of a deep, pervasive, and volatile set of social sentiments. These sentiments do not have to be inherently related but can become integrated through the activities of the strategically situated individual or group. Hence, existential-conflict theorists do not discount the work of labelling theorists but rather investigate an area that the latter have glossed over. The moral entrepreneur is significant not because he generates public sentiment against the drug user but because he coordinates and integrates enough public sentiment, from whatever source, to implement the passage of his desired legislation. Hence, the existential-conflict theorists place the moral entrepreneur at the gate of the legal process. They also move easily beyond this point to the existential basis for the public support that flows through this gate and into the seat of political power; that is, they also address the larger structural tensions pervasive throughout society.

Although this approach is rather recent, it finds considerable support in one of the classic works on the dynamics of anti-intoxicant legislation. During the 1950s, Gusfield did a classic study of the temperance movement, a study that has addressed a number of issues I have discussed. Although Gusfield's work falls within the domain of more traditional sociological research, its conclusions are not dissimilar to mine presented in this book. These issues include the need for theoretical flexibility between the microlevel and macrolevel, the interface of emotions and cognitions in forming a social definition or label, the importance of structural tensions in creating the emotions supporting a label, and the structure of the information feedback loops that result from these factors.

Gusfield's work is grounded in the social reality of "real people, in real places, and the writing or artifacts that they have made." Through interviews and archival studies of the documents produced by the Women's Christian Temperance Union, influential political figures, and other prohibitionist groups, Gusfield was able to move from the existential base reflected in these interviews and artifacts toward an understanding of the larger social tensions that motivated this anti-intoxicant movement. Through the close scrutiny of the experiences of those who took part in this movement, he discerned a complex structure of feelings that came together to generate the temperance movement. He found that the existential reality he had uncovered did not fit easily into the prevailing theoretical categories of traditional sociology. The study of the rise and fall of the Volstead Act, which outlawed the manufacturing and distribution of alcohol, is an example of social movements that cannot be placed precisely in cognitive (instrumental) or emotional (expressive) terms. "Most movements, and most political acts, contain a mixture of instrumental, expressive, and symbolic elements ... those issues which have appeared as 'matters of principle' now appear to us to be related to status conflicts and are understandable in symbolic terms."[13] Here the social movements to control the use of alcohol can be seen not as a purely instrumental attempt to control potentially antisocial behavior but rather as a law that represents deep emotions of fear, frustration, and mistrust on the part of a declining social group. The rural middle class, whose ideals of hard work, piety, and sobriety dominated the United States, faced a cultural confrontation by the turn of this century. Although these values had enjoyed relative hegemony since the Revolutionary War, they were being eclipsed by the more earthy values of immediate gratification, physical pleasure, and uncontrolled intoxication on the part of the rising urban working class. Along with industrialization came waves of European immigrants who congregated in the cities and grew in numbers, visibility, and political clout. As Gusfield noted, "Precisely because drinking and non-drinking have been ways to identify the members of a subculture, drinking and abstinence became symbols of social status, identifying social levels of the society whose styles of life separated them culturally."[14] The Volstead Act was a symbolic reflection of deep-seated emotions on the part of the middle classes that had become fused with an instrumental attempt to place legal sanctions on behavior they considered reprehensible. Because Gusfield's study focused on the existential base of this movement, he acknowledged the need to move beyond the traditional categories used to interpret this behavior. He wrote, "Between instrumental and expressive politics there is no bin into which the symbolic goals of status movements can be analytically placed. Our usage of symbolic politics is an effort to provide such a bin."[15]

Not only does his work reflect theoretical flexibility; it also addresses the central issue of the role of emotions and cognitions in the formation of this social definition:

> Moral fervor does not happen in a vacuo apart from a specific setting. We [have to examine] the social conditions which made the fact of other people's drinking especially galling to the abstainer and the need for reformist actions...these conditions are found in the development of threats to the socially dominant position of the Temperance adherent by those whose style of life differs from his.[16]

It was not drinking that put the real force behind the movement to control intoxicants; it was the emotional contamination of this issue with the much more powerful feelings of fear and frustration encountered when one's entire cultural edifice comes under attack. Neither drinking nor drug use is significant enough in itself to warrant a massive legislative movement. Rather, it is the fluid nature of human emotions and their transformation into simple labels or categories that enables an individual or group to manipulate this transformational process into a symbolic crusade.

These diffuse feelings were the result of large-scale and long-term structural tensions stemming from the industrial revolution. Along with the rise of major industrial centers in the Northeast after the Civil War came a tremendous influx of immigrants, poor rural Americans, and drifters. And as their demographic concentration increased, they became more visible politically and socially. The position one took on the issue of temperance "was one of the ways society could distinguish the industrious from the ne'er-do-well; the steady worker from the unreliable drifter, the good credit risk from the bad gamble; the native American from the immigrant."[17] With the pervasive structural shifts taking place during the late nineteenth century, many found refuge in the simplicity of the temperance issue, thus not having to face the complexity of their changing world.

Not only does Gusfield's study provide insight into the role of large structural tensions in the formation of the emotional and cognitive complex that constitutes the core symbol of the social movement, but his findings also allude to an information feedback loop. His study does not explicitly address the existence of such a loop, but his general findings fit well with that theoretical notion. Specifically, he found that the temperance movement represented a desire to dominate, at least symbolically, the cultures of those whom native, rural, Protestant Americans considered objectionable. This process of status domination, or subcultural alienation, to use Hess's term, implies that "public support of one conception of morality at the expense of another enhances the prestige and self-esteem of the victors and degrades the culture of the losers."[18] Hence, as with Hess's work on the rise of drug laws, the feedback loop not only defines users of intoxicants as deviant, but it necessarily elevates the status of nonusers. As this loop is politically manipulated to gain the emotional infusion from other, usually unrelated issues, the loop expands and becomes the basis for legislative sanctions.

Thus, Gusfield's study on intoxicants clearly expands beyond the limitations of the labelling perspective to address the complex role of emotions and cognitions, the influences of large, structural tensions, and, implicitly, the effect of these variables on the structuring of a feedback loop. His work, however, only focuses on one side of the legal process: the interplay between the social order and the rise of legislative sanctions. The other aspect of this process concerns the role of law enforcement agencies in their attempts to fulfill the legislative mandate to control the use of intoxicants. It is this area that I focus on in most of this book.

Once the mandate has been passed, a formal organization—in this case the Federal Bureau of Narcotics—is formed to enforce it. Just as the moral entrepreneur acts as a mediator between the social order and the legal mandate, so the law enforcement agencies mediate back from the specific law to its practical impact on the social order. In both cases, the manipulation and control of information is the central aspect of gaining and maintaining power and effectiveness. Whereas the moral entrepreneur manipulates information on a number of levels to gain the passage of legislation—for example, at conferences, in the mass media, and at congressional hearings—so too the law enforcement agents focus on this aspect of acquiring power. Law enforcement agencies manipulate information in Congress too, but they also have significant forms of information control both within themselves and in the field where suspects are apprehended.

Chapter 1 of this book discusses the social factors that gave rise to the antidrug legislation. Chapter 2 focuses on the role of information control within the Federal Bureau of Narcotics (FBN) and how it manipulates legal ambiguities to increase its organizational power. Special attention is paid to the strategies the FBN uses to control the definition of drug abuse, expand its jurisdiction over other drugs, and use different crises to buttress its image as an effective law enforcement agency. The existential-conflict perspective, especially the theoretical work by Collins on organizational structures, is very useful in the elucidation of this process. Just as was the case with the rise of the initial antidrug legislation, the initial role of the bureau was not clearly defined and, hence, problematic. However, the bureau and its leadership were politically astute enough to realize that their organization had to become a symbol of effective antidrug administration. To achieve this cognitive image, they effectively manipulated the definition of the legal mandate against drug abuse, integrated class and racial tensions behind the antidrug perspective, and created strong political ties with key congressional powers. Through these and other strategies, the FBN was able to dominate the cognitive image of the drug addict, coalesce public emotions behind the bureau organization, and expand its legal jurisdiction to a larger domain of intoxicants. With the implementation of each new strategy, the FBN expanded and refined the negative feedback loop between the drug user and the public as a whole. Whether it is the moral entrepreneur or the organizational bureaucrat who wants to expand this social definition and, hence his power, it is the control of information that makes this process successful.

Chapters 3 and 4 are concerned with the practical enforcement procedures used by the criminal justice system to enforce the antidrug laws. Here again, the existential-conflict theory is seen to move easily from a macrosocial to a microinteractional context. Of special concern in these chapters is the divergent strategies of the U.S. Customs, which is primarily responsible for drug interdiction along the international border, and that of the FBN's newest organizational progeny, the Drug Enforcement Administration (DEA), an outgrowth of the FBN now responsible for drug enforcement in both the national and international domains. There has been some intense conflict between this agency and the more established Customs, a conflict that has significantly reduced the effectiveness of both groups.

The analysis of the control of information presented in the first two chapters is central to the remaining chapters, which explore not only the conflict between these two groups concerning how information is to be generated and disseminated among law enforcement agencies, but also how it is used within the practical field activities of their respective agents. Here too, the interface between cognitions and emotions is of central importance to organizational power. Customs has generated a relatively effective system for screening suspects and generating legally sound cases at the ports of entry along the international borders. The agents' ability to control the situational context at these ports enables them to create an information feedback loop through which suspects can be identified and apprehended. Specifically, agents control information in a manner that generates an emotional response by the suspect, which then becomes grounds for a solid court case. Thus, the emotional content of a situation is the existential basis on which the cognitive and, hence, legal structure is generated.

This is also true in the work of the DEA when generating information while plea bargaining their cases. Whereas the Customs agents focus their attention on the ports of entry to curtail drug traffic into this country, the DEA has emphasized the pressuring of defendants to divulge information during plea negotiations. Through this information, DEA officials believe that they can can set up and apprehend other, more important, drug smugglers. Again, the manipulation of the situation in a way that generates the desired emotional response— in this case within the defendant—is the key to organizational success. The basic strategy of the DEA, like that of the moral entrepreneur and Customs, is the effective control of information within problematic social situations.

FUNCTIONALIST THEORY: THE LAW AS A MEANS OF SOCIAL INTEGRATION?

Although this analysis argues that the existential-conflict perspective is the most fruitful in elucidating the salient elements of the drug issue, one other theoretical perspective must be addressed. Although the functionalist perspective has not contributed to the drug literature in a major way, it has had a significant impact on the sociological tradition as a whole, and thus its relevance to this issue must be examined.

Like the macroconflict theorists, the functionalists see the law as reflecting deeply held social emotions. However, unlike the existential-conflict theorists, the functionalists assume that the law facilitates the integration of various groups within the society, clearly demarcates the collectively held values of the social order, and assures stable and patterned interaction among the members of society. Where the conflict theorists see the law as a tool of domination, functionalists assume it is a means of integration. Where the conflict theorists see social values as essentially problematic and unresolved, functionalists assume value consensus. Where the conflict theorists see the law as ensuring the imposition of the dominant group's norms on a minority, the functionalists see it as ensuring mutually beneficial and coordinated interaction. The functionalists tend to focus on the social order as a whole and give little, if any, attention to the interaction of individuals in everyday life. Hence, this perspective is relevant only for chapter 1 on the rise of societal-wide, antidrug legislation. Irrespective of the inherent limitations of the functionalist view in addressing all aspects of the drug issue, its importance within the sociological tradition requires that it be given consideration in those areas where it is relevant. Thus, its contribution and limitations will be spelled out, along with the more useful theoretical paradigms in chapter 1.

1 PEOPLE AND PROBLEMATIC MEANINGS: THE EXISTENTIAL EFFECTS, SOCIAL CONTEXTS, AND CLASS CONFLICT SURROUNDING DRUG USE

In the late nineteenth century, the United States was beginning its evolution from a rural, sparsely inhabited, commercial society toward the present densely populated, urban, and industrial society. During this period, public perception concerning the proper use of drugs (opiates, cocaine, and marijuana) began to change significantly. What was initially an area governed by personal preference and subcultural norms has come increasingly under the control of legal sanctions. Although there has never been a universal consensus as to the legitimacy of the laws governing the use of drugs for personal pleasure, there have been an increasing number of legislative guidelines designed to control and eliminate drug use for nonmedical purposes.

Along with the rise of a more complex and differentiated social order came a diversity of perspectives on the proper role of drugs. The inherently problematic nature of the effects of drugs on users allowed for significant variation in the meanings imputed to drug use. These imputed meanings varied not only within each particular drug episode experienced by users, but there was also considerable disparity among members of a given class and, most importantly, a major conflict between classes. Some men of letters, including Baudelaire and De Quincey, used opium to increase their artistic and imaginative capacities. Middle-class women used opium and cocaine for medicinal purposes, either in the form of a prescription from a physician or in one of the numerous patent medicines available without a prescription. In the cities on the West Coast, especially San Francisco, Chinese immigrants smoked opium to relieve the tensions of their arduous labor in small factories and on the railroads. In the South, blacks were thought to use cocaine in soft drinks and for medicinal purposes. And in the Southwest, Mexican immigrants were prone to use marijuana for their personal pleasure after working in the vegetable fields and fruit orchards. Whether they were middle or lower class, white or an ethnic minority, men of artistic talent or just everyday citizens, a significant number of people in the United States used drugs from around 1860 to 1915.

The most vivid existential descriptions of the subjective effects of drugs are presented by nineteenth-century writers whose gift for colorful descriptions made their experiences a natural existential point of departure for the understanding of the fundamental feelings involved in drug use. From this point, it is possible to analyze the way different sectors of the social order constructed, imputed, and disseminated information about drug use that developed into feedback loops.

THE MEDICAL CONTEXT FOR DRUG USE: ECSTASY AND TERROR AMONG THE MIDDLE CLASSES

Members of the middle class who used drugs, usually opium or its derivatives, were often introduced to them through the professional recommendations of a physician. One of the most open and celebrated groups to contact drugs in this manner were men of letters. Although the positive meaning of drug use was initially determined by the medical context in which it was prescribed, the subjective realities of the drug experience were often less than medicinal.

In England, Thomas De Quincey took laudanum, opium in an alcohol solution, on the advice of his doctor to relieve rheumatic pains in his head. His classic *Confessions of an English Opium Eater*, written in 1821, described the psychological effects of the drug. He wrote:

That my pains had vanished was now a trifle in my eyes; this negative effect was swallowed up in the immensity of those positive effects which had opened up before me, in the abyss of divine enjoyment thus suddenly revealed. Here was a panacea...here was the secret of happiness, about which philosophers had disputed for so many ages, at once discovered; happiness might now be bought for a penny.[1]

But as he continued to experiment with the drug for personal rather than medicinal purposes, "the full terror of one's imagination and dreams" also became apparent. Toward the end of his *Confessions*, De Quincey wrote:

I fled from the wrath of Brama through all the forests of Asia; Vishnu hated me: Seeva laid wait for me.... I was buried, for a thousand years, in stone coffins, with mummies and sphinxes, in narrow chambers at the heart of eternal pyramids. I was kissed, with cancerous kisses, by crocodiles; and laid, confounded with all unutterable slimy things, amongst reeds and Nilotic mud.[2]

De Quincey, and later Baudelaire, appreciated the multifaceted effects that drugs could have on users. They felt that opium acted as an agent to intensify the dream proclivities laying dormant in each individual. As *Confessions* indicates, these dreams could be "the secret of happiness" or the full terror of exotic eastern gods bent on one's destruction.

Although De Quincey was read in the United States, the most significant public statement on the effects of opium by an American was William Blair's *An Opium-Eater in America* (1825). Like De Quincey, Blair first ingested the drug for primarily medicinal reasons but soon became engrossed in the existential effects. Blair was a man of weak physical stature and had spent several years of his youth absorbed in books and mental activity. This led to a collapse of most of his physical strength and prompted him to turn to opium for "artificial stimuli [to] obtain a sudden increase in strength."[3] He felt this stimulus was necessary for him to maintain his job as a clerk to which he was unfit by "habit, inclination, and constitution."[4]

Like De Quincey, he found his solution to be double edged. After taking the drug with coffee, he felt a growing increase in strength and a "gradual creeping thrill...inducing a sensation of dreamy exhilaration...similar in nature but not in degree to the drowsiness caused by wine, though not inclining me to sleep;...I longed to engage in some active exercise; to sing, dance, or leap."[5] He went to the theater, where he was plunged into pleasures and visions of "Titanian splendor and immensity."[6] The stage and actors seemed to disappear, and he was confronted by endless corridors and galleries, each stretched out with magnificent gems and refracting lights. His feelings of elation continued after the theater, and on the road home he "knocked down...the first watchman [he] met: of course there was 'a row.'"[7]

Several hours later at home, the other side of the drug made itself manifest. Blair had read De Quincey's description of the positive effects of opium, but of the miseries of opium he "had most unaccountably neglected to read."[8] Although he had not read De Quincey's description, he gave a vivid account of the after-effects himself:

My misery commenced. Burning heat, attended with constant thirst, then began to torment me from morning till night: my skin became scurfy; the skin of my feet and hands peeled off; my tongue was always furred; a feeling of contraction in the bowels was continual; my eyes were strained and discolored, and I had unceasing head-ache.[9]

As Hess suggests, these descriptions of the different effects of drug use can become the foundations for either a positive or a negative feedback loop. Should information begin to circulate that reflects the "misery," "burning heat," or hallucination of one's "skin peeling off," the voluntary drug user would immediately begin to be perceived as less than reasonable. Hess argues that it was these poets and writers who first popularized drug use and initiated the negative circulation of information concerning its effects. However, the medical context in which the drug was prescribed and the salient social support that existed for the medical profession staved off this definition for a good part of the nineteenth century. It would take more than poetic descriptions to arouse enough public sentiment to countermand the medical profession's positive definition of drug use.

With the invention of the hypodermic needle and its introduction to America in 1856, the medical profession saw the injection of opium intravenously as a cornerstone for the alleviation of pain.[10] This idea received significant support during the Civil War when thousands of soldiers were given morphine to reduce the pain from wounds and subsequent surgery. Medical journals of the day were replete with glowing descriptions of the effectiveness of the drug during wartime and its obvious advantages for peacetime medical practice. Because the medical profession was concerned with developing a professional image that reflected knowledgeable and effective means for alleviating physical suffering, its members tended to circulate positive claims made about these drugs. This, coupled with the public's desire for simple cures for complex physical ailments, put considerable pressure on physicians to provide a simple, if biased, view concerning the effects of these drugs. Thus although the negative effects of the drug were noticed by some researchers, the medical profession chose not to incorporate these factors into the social context of prescribing drugs.

Of the negative findings on opium use, one of the first concerned a longitudinal study of Civil War veterans. Following the Civil War, many soldiers who had come in contact with morphine continued to use it and became addicted. Their addiction became known as the "army disease," and there were still many afflicted by it at the turn of the century. One researcher of conditions in homes for retired veterans commented:

Many veterans of the Civil War became morphinists to relieve the pain and suffering following injuries received in the service.... The sufferings and hardships growing out of the perils of war often react in illness, nerve and brain instability, and feebleness, and the use of morphine is a symptom of damage from this source.[11]

In spite of this evidence and other studies conducted at this time, respected and reputable doctors commonly prescribed a reasonable amount of morphine to a patient suffering from a chronic or incurable ailment or from postoperative pain. Given the often busy schedule of the physician, it was common practice to leave the syringe and drug with the family to be administered in case of increased pain. Because there were no legal restrictions on the drug's usage, a patient would often increase the amount and/or number of injections per day. It did not take long for these individuals to become addicted.

The problem of morphine addiction was especially prevalent among middle-aged women. Given the chronic types of ailments afflicting women during this period of life—such as child bearing, pelvic inflammations, rheumatism, neuralgia, arthritis, and, most importantly, painful menstruation—doctors commonly prescribed opiates for a considerable period of time and on a regular basis. Again, the doctor would often leave the syringe and prescription for the drug with the patient or her family, and the patient could easily fill the prescription as many times as she felt necessary. It was a small step from the simple alleviation of a chronically painful ailment to addiction. The studies conducted between 1880 and 1924 indicate that approximately 60 percent of the cases occurred among morphine addiction were middle-aged women.

A related problem involved the addiction of babies, either because the mother was addicted at the time of the birth or because morphine was given to soothe a crying child. A physician at New York University indicated that as early as 1832, many a "youthful, inconsiderate mother and the idle nurse, too frequently resort to opium to hush the infant's cries."[12] This fear was confirmed, much later, in 1903 by the American Pharmaceutical Association, which stated that it had received many reports from both pharmacists and physicians indicating that mothers were addicting their infants through breast feeding or by giving them opiated syrups.

Although men were not the typical morphine addicts, they were still susceptible to addiction if the social context was conducive. They would become addicted after taking morphine to reduce some physical ailment, but they were motivated more commonly to procure the drug to reduce mental and emotional tensions due to occupational stress, often the result of being overworked and of psychic tensions stemming from a competetive middle-class work ethic. One representative study conducted by the American Pharmaceutical Association describes the cause of morphine addiction in men of the upper and middle classes:

Society's whirl demands late hours—a little punch, perhaps salad; sleep must be immediate or the man of business will not get any . . . the man of business must develop the idea which is to yield an extra profit quickly, gain the advantage over his competitor; this may make him nervous, but what of it? That can be remedied by the physician.[13]

The busy schedule and resulting nervous tension, insomnia, and irritability made individuals less effective in their daily life. To alleviate these symptoms, many men would turn to the relaxing effects of morphine and the various over-the-counter remedies containing morphine.

Ironically much evidence indicates that physicians themselves were the victims of their own prescriptions. Doctors were not only concerned with occupational success but also had direct access to the drugs. Their lax attitude toward prescribing the drugs to patients was reflected in their tendency to use the drug to relieve their own physical pains and tensions.

By the turn of the century, however, the negative effects of opiates had become visible enough for the more sensitive members of the medical profession to look for a new means of reducing the pain of opium addiction. The medical profession began to try to restructure its doctor-patient information loops. Although there was notable effort to constrain the indiscriminate use of opiates within the medical context, little effort was made to reevaluate a key assumption within the profession's view on drugs. Specifically, the profession reaffirmed what Douglas has termed "the Pollyanna assumption about drugs [or] . . . the principle of substituting a secret problem for a publicized one."[14] If the addictive characteristics of the opiates had become a well-publicized problem, the medical profession set out to find a new, lesser-known drug to replace it. Retaining the assumptions that drugs are the best means for attaining medical objectives, the profession began to expand the positive circulation of information on a new drug, cocaine.

Sigmund Freud was a pioneer in the use of cocaine and was interested in its therapeutic aspects for opium addiction, especially in relation to his personal friend, Dr. Fleischl, a morphine addict. He gave a small dose to Fleischl and found that it had a positive and immediate effect. Fleischl hated the way that morphine dulled his senses and mental acuity and is said to have clutched at the new drug like a drowning man and within a few days was taking it continually. These results prompted Freud to experiment with cocaine himself to relieve the depression, fatigue, and other neurotic problems that had plagued him for years. Upon taking the drug, Freud found that it created

exhilaration and lasting euphoria, which in no way differs from the normal euphoria of the healthy person. . . . You perceive an increase of self-control and possess more vitality and capacity for work. . . . In other words, you are simply normal, and it is soon hard to believe that you are under the influence of any drug.[15]

Freud's description could easily be integrated into the middle-class ideal of self-control and hard work, as well as the medical context of effective pain relief. If the deadening and lethargic effects of opium use could be overcome by taking cocaine instead and the effects were simply to make the individual more vigorous, the medical profession could spread the word of this wonder drug. Indeed contemporary medical research revealed considerable agreement within the profession on the therapeutic effects of cocaine for opium addiction.

In spite of this early optimism, Freud and other members of the profession soon found the existential reality of cocaine use to be problematic. Within a year, Freud's friend Fleischl had increased his intake of cocaine to one gram a day, a hundred times the quantity Freud was accustomed to taking. This immoderate use of cocaine led Fleischl into acute cocaine poisoning with psychotic reactions in which he saw "white snakes creeping over his skin."[16] Fleischl's reaction greatly disturbed Freud, but he felt that the drug still had therapeutic value if taken in moderation. Freud was aware of the effects of very large doses of cocaine—eventual convulsions, symptoms of paralysis and death due to paralysis of the respiratory system—from his review of the experiments done on animals but still attempted to reconcile these effects with his initially positive label. To do this, he reverted to a major cornerstone of the middle-class value system: the strong and independent will. Freud argued not that the use of cocaine was inherently detrimental but that it was individuals with a weak will who were most susceptible to a negative reaction. He claimed, based on his own experience with Fleischl, that all

reports of addiction to cocaine and deterioration resulting from it refer to morphine addicts, persons who, already in the grip of one demon are so weak in willpower, so susceptible, that they would misuse, and indeed have misused, any stimulant held out to them. Cocaine has claimed no other, no victim on its own.[17]

Here Freud attempted to revitalize his positive definition of cocaine use by infusing it with one of the simplest and most salient aspects of middle-class morality. Based on evidence gathered since the Civil War, Freud was willing to contribute to the circulation of negative information on the effects of opium, but he was not willing to recognize the problematic aspects of cocaine use and attempted to strike a positive emotional cord with the middle-class medical profession to bolster his definition and, possibly, his career. In Freud's view, strong-willed individuals could reap benefits from this powerful stimulant. However, the effects of morphine were so devastating that it could cripple this moral component within the individual and make him "susceptible...to the misuse" of this new drug.

Although Freud did not recognize it, he had touched on a key feature of the moral definition that would be used to sanction drug use in the early 1900s. The ideal of a strong and unencumbered will has been central to the middle-class system of values—values that emphasize self-discipline, hard work, and productivity. The social sentiments surrounding the notion of possibly losing this psychological foundation are deep, pervasive, and powerful. Evidence indicates that Freud did not hesitate to use this fact. However, in the long run, Freud's efforts to solidify a positive definition of cocaine use within the profession and, possibly within the larger society, did not materialize. Not being particularly weak-willed himself, he turned from the problematics of chemical cures for human ailments to the equally problematic area of psychological cures. As Freud's work indicates, there was considerable uncertainty as to the value of these two drugs for medical purposes, a degree of uncertainty that would last until the second decade of this century. The life and tribulations of another physician, Dr. William Halsted, reflects this time period well.

Cocaine was introduced to America by Dr. William Halsted, a man often described as the Father of Modern Surgery. Halsted used cocaine in a much wider context than did Freud and found that it could produce a nerve block in almost any area of the body, making it a versatile and, he believed, safe local anesthetic. He wrote several papers on the subject in 1885 and was not heard from for almost a year. Like many researchers of the day, after having experimented on animals, he tried the drug himself and became habituated to it. He was finally able to stop taking cocaine after a number of trips to different hospitals, but only by taking up morphine as a replacement. Although a morphine addict from 1886 until his death, some thirty-eight years later at the age of seventy, he was able to complete a brilliant medical career.

Although Halsted's experiences should have been a source of caution in the medical and pharmacological industries, the positive moral context of the medicinal use of these drugs successfully precluded such a response. Between 1885 and 1906, medical practitioners, pharmacists, and the patent medicine industry all advertised and sold cocaine and products containing cocaine as new wonder drugs. Freud and others had expounded cocaine as a therapeutic drug for morphine addiction, Halsted had demonstrated its use as a local anesthetic, and now various entrepreneurs in Europe and America were about to make it a wonder drug for all physical and mental ailments or a means of increasing one's vigor and vitality. During this period, literally hundreds of remedies on the market contained cocaine, and many of them still survive today, although without the cocaine. The most well-known is Coca-Cola, which contained cocaine for seventeen years (1886-1903). In 1903 when law forbade including the cocaine the manufacturer replaced it with caffeine, which it hoped would be similar. Although Coca-Cola is the most well known, there were many imitators during its initial heyday. According to the American Medical Association's booklet, *Nostrums and Quackery* (1912), cocaine could be found in a number of soft drinks: "Kos-Kola, Kola-Ade, Koca-Nola, Cafe-Coca Compound, Pillsbury's Coke Extract, Celery Cola, Coke Extract, Dr. Don's Kola, Vani-Kola Compound Syrup, Rococola, and Wiseola."[18] What had started as a medical wonder drug and had enjoyed an initial moral insulation within the context of the medical profession was rapidly circulating into the larger society. With this spread came increased tension concerning the proper social interpretation of the use of these drugs, a tension reflected in the popular literature of the day.

Sir Arthur Conan Doyle's character, Sherlock Holmes, used cocaine between investigations, and his close friend, Doctor Watson, was often instrumental in procuring and administering the drug. However, as within medical circles, there seems to have been considerable confusion about the actual effects of this drug. The first mention of cocaine by Doyle was in *Scandal in Bohemia*, published in 1886, in which Holmes is characterized as "alternating from week to week between cocaine and ambition, the drowsiness of the drug and the fierce energy of his own keen nature."[19] Doyle indicates that Holmes would have to rise "out of his drug-created dreams, and [become] hot upon the scent of some new problem."[20] Although Doyle was trained as a physician, he seems to have confused the effects of cocaine with those of opium and morphine. Instead of the "exhilaration and lasting euphoria, which in no way differs from the normal euphoria of the healthy person" described by Freud, Holmes was described as drowsy, and the drug was antithetical to his own keen nature. However, Doyle changed his view of cocaine two years later, perhaps after his personal experimentation. In *The Sign of the Four*, he described Holmes's use of cocaine as "transcendingly stimulating and clarifying to the mind that its secondary action is a matter of small amount."[21] Although he had become aware of the normal stimulating effects of cocaine, he was also becoming aware of its other possible effects: physical weakening and possible paranoid delusions. In some of the later novels, such as *The Final Problem*, Doyle describes Holmes as much paler and weaker from the use of the drug and exhibiting some classic paranoid fantasies about his arch rival, Moriarty.

If the effects of the opiates and cocaine were an unresolved issue in the popular mind, this was no less the case with the third controversial drug: marijuana. As in the case of the other two drugs, the literary descriptions of the drug were highly ambivalent. The French poet, Baudelaire, wrote in his classic *Les pardis artificels* that the drug could transform the mortal personality of the user to "a final, supreme thought [which] bursts from the dreamers brain: 'I have become God.'"[22] However, during more sedate moments, he suggested that hashish, a derivative of or marijuana, is "nothing miraculous, absolutely nothing but an exaggeration of the natural. The brain and organism on which it operates will produce only the normal phenomena particular to that individual—increase, admittedly in number and force, but always faithful to their origin."[23] Baudelaire remained true to the existential reality of drug use, which suggested that the effects of the drug, when viewed from the subjective experiences of the user, were highly individualized. Each individual brought a unique quality to the experience, a quality that made it difficult to develop consistent generalizations concerning its effects on the user.

If Baudelaire recognized the existential nature of the drug, he was also sensitive to the middle-class values of an unencumbered will and its centrality to a moral interpretation of drug use. He warned of the possible result of using this chemical source of knowledge too often. "Later on, perhaps, a too frequent consultation of the oracle will diminish your strength of will; perhaps you will be less of a man than you are today."[24] Although some investigators feel that his fear of losing will power was probably due more to his previous experiences with opium, this theme was reiterated by another influential person, Bayard Taylor.

Taylor, an American, was called the Laureate of the Gilded Age and was well known for his poetry, novels, and government service as secretary of American litigation in St. Petersburg, Russia, and Germany. Widely traveled and with a popular following, Taylor, like others who had experimented with the drug, described "thrills which ran through my nervous system ... accompanied with sensations that steeped my whole being in unutterable rapture."[25] Taylor gave vivid accounts of his fantasies, which related to the places he had experienced: "I suddenly found myself at the foot of the great Pyramid of Cheops ... [which] gleamed like gold in the sun ... gorgeous fancies of the Arabian Nights ... Mrs. Browning's 'Rhyme of the Duchess May' flashed into my mind."[26] More importantly, like Baudelaire and others, he was concerned with his apparent loss of will caused by the drug: "The remnant of will with which I struggled against the demon [drug], became gradually weaker, and I felt that I should too be powerless in his hands. Every effort to preserve my reason was accompanied by a pang of mortal fear, lest what I now experienced was insanity, and would hold master over me for ever."[27] After the effects of the drug had worn off, Taylor vowed to abstain from the drug in the future. However, he did not regret taking the drug because he felt that it made him aware of the majesty of human reason and of human will, even at its weakest, and the awful peril of tampering with that which assails their integrity. This was a lesson that he was determined to convey to others by means of antidrug legislation. Taylor was just one of many Americans who were interested in furthering this moral orientation toward drug use by creating legal sanctions.

Like opium and cocaine, marijuana enjoyed a brief career as a wonder drug used with the moral shield of the medical profession.

Some found that it could be used to relieve the pains of opiate withdrawal, a conclusion confirmed in the late nineteenth century and fifty years later in a New York City study sponsored by Mayor Fiorello La Guardia. This study reported, "I am satisfied of its immense value [in withdrawing patients from opiates]... the chief point that struck me was the immediate action of the drug in appeasing the appetite for the ... opium and restoring the ability to appreciate food."[28] The La Guardia Report (1938) also explored the relation between cannabis and opiate addiction and found that in both opiate and alcohol intoxication, cannabis was effective in relieving much of the pain and tension of withdrawal.

Although many researchers were interested in the medicinal effects of cannabis, it soon became apparent that this use had serious problems. Although it lacked the addictive effects of the opiates, it was difficult to synthesize the drug into a constant potency because of variations in the ripeness, humidity, soil characteristics, and temperature in which the plants had been grown.

The most important drawback of the drug was the problematic reaction of different people to the same dosage. J. R. Reynolds, an astute clinician in the 1880s, observed that "individuals differ widely in their relations to many medicines and articles of diet especially those of vegetable origin—such as ... cannabis."[29] By the turn of the century cannabis was stricken from the list of medical drugs as numerous tranquilizers and relaxants whose dosage and potency could be accurately gauged were discovered and synthesized. The medical community turned to these drugs because of their lower cost and perceived predictability.

The existential reality of drug use by members of the middle class in the nineteenth and early twentieth centuries reveals a number of similarities among the three most commonly used drugs—opium, cocaine, and marijuana. The essentially problematic nature of these drugs created conflicting interpretations as to their effects by members of the middle class, men of letters, and even within the medical profession. Opium, cocaine, and, to a lesser extent, marijuana enjoyed an initially positive definition due to the medical context in which they were prescribed, but a lack of control over their dissemination within this context and a tendency to ignore the negative effects allowed addiction and/or negative psychological reactions to spread. In spite of this, the medical profession legitimated the use of these drugs to a degree that assured the dominance of a positive definition of their effects for most of the nineteenth century.

In the case of opium, a positive feedback loop between doctors and patients had developed, which spread to nonusers who were eager to ameliorate their personal ailments with this drug. As demand increased, the pharmaceutical companies met these needs with over-the-counter syrups, sedatives to calm tense males, pills to relieve the females suffering from painful menstruation, and even formulas to stop crying children. Although the negative effects of the drug were known since De Quincey's time and more sensitive members of the medical profession questioned its indiscriminate use, the positive medical definition remained strong until around the turn of the century.

Although cocaine did not have as long a medical career, it did enjoy much of the same, initially positive, support that was afforded to opium. It too was billed as a drug that could relieve the burden of human suffering—even the suffering of opium addiction. Its potential negative effects did not deter the rise of the drug in numerous products consumed by the public. However, in spite of the medical profession's tendency to indulge in the Pollyanna principle, the negative effects were eventually recognized.

Marijuana did not enjoy the same degree of support that the medical profession afforded to opium and cocaine. Because it was a drug used primarily by Mexicans and became available after the antidrug movement was on the rise (1910), it did not have the same expansive positive feedback loop. However, some members of the medical profession did discuss its potential for relieving the problem of opiate addiction. Although it did not enjoy the legitimating context of medical use, it ultimately received the same structural treatment that caused the other two drugs to become the focus of extremely negative legal sanctions. The reasons for the dominance of the negative over the initially positive definitions of these drugs lie within the shifting tensions of class conflict.

THE REPREHENSIBLE CONTEXT OF DRUG USE: THE OSTRACISM AND OPPRESSION OF MINORITIES

If drug use was introduced to the middle class within the legitimating context of the physician-patient relationship, its use by members

of certain highly visible minorities—Chinese, blacks, and Chicanos—
did not benefit from such forms of social insulation. Given this lack of
a clear legitimating context, drug use among the lower classes was
open to severe, negative, moral interpretations by those who wielded
power and influence. This vulnerability made lower-class drug users a
natural symbol through which larger economic, social, and political
tensions could be focused. Just as Gusfield found middle- and lower-
class tensions focused on the temperance issue, so did similar tensions
become vented in the drug problem.

The symbolic structure of the antidrug campaign revolved around
the image of "the dope fiend," a term that first appeared in the *New
York Sun* in 1896. Although this was the first formal appearance of
this term, its content had been generated and expanded over the
several decades that preceded the turn of the century. There were a
number of attributes imputed into this symbol, but three stand out as
the most salient in creating the emotional climate necessary for the
passage of antidrug legislation. Whereas the middle-class user was
assumed to have taken the drug for medicinal purposes, the drug
fiend was seen as desiring, even craving, only its pleasurable effects.
Further, the drug user often required ever more powerful pleasures
and tended to expand his desires from relatively innocuous stimulants, like cigarettes, toward the addictive drugs. One journalist wrote
that "the relationship of tabacco, especially in the form of cigarettes,
and alcohol and opium is a very close one. Morphine is the legitimate
consequence of tobacco. Cigarettes, drink, and opium is the logical
and regular series."[30] Finally, this uncontrolled desire for more exotic
pleasures necessarily weakened the individual's will and the lower,
more bestial forces of lust and rage were certain to become unleashed.

These three attributes, which created the image of the dope fiend,
fit well with some very real social, economic, and political fears felt by
the middle class during this period. Along with increased industrialization came an ever-increasing propinquity between the middle and
lower classes. Prior to this time, the middle class had enjoyed relative
hegemony and a degree of clear differentiation from the lower class.
However, as both groups became more dependent on the rising urban
industrial economy and the closer proximity that city living entailed,
the barriers began to disintegrate. The lower class, which had been
relegated to a position across the tracks, was becoming more numerous and more visible. This increased propinquity implied the possibil-

ity of moral contamination. If the dope fiend initially began to crave more lascivious pleasure by first starting with innocuous cigarettes, it was not inconceivable that these individuals could entice respectable citizens with the same, seemingly innocent, start. The need to isolate this threat seemed obvious.

This desire to isolate the dope fiend had economic and political underpinnings. Although the drug addict, whether minority or middle class, was not a large enough population to be a major factor in the economy, certain minority groups did pose such a threat. Chinese made up a significant sector of the economy in the West; blacks threatened white interests in the South; and Mexicans represented a major economic force in the Southwest. Although the demographic, economic, and cultural tensions differed somewhat with each minority group, they all became seen as a group that threatened the dominant white society. As such, it was natural that there would be a movement to isolate and legally dominate them. Antidrug legislation provided one symbolic avenue toward this end. The reality of these structural tensions ultimately provided the emotional momentum necessary to ensure the spread of the negative definition of drug use among the nondrug users, the stabilization of that feedback loop, and ultimately the political foundations for the moral entrepreneur.

Chinese and Anti-Opium Legislation

The first antinarcotics legislation, passed in the urban areas of the West, was designed to protect the respectable classes against a foreign influence—in this case, the Chinese. The Chinese immigrated to California in the 1850s to work the newly discovered goldfields. Because of the destruction resulting from the Tai Ping Revolution (1850E1864), and the serious flooding in the southeastern provinces of China in the early 1850s, many Chinese hoped to find the wealth in America that would enable them to get a fresh start here or permit them to return to their native land. After the goldfields were played out by the early 1870s, these immigrants went to work on the railroads, in small businesses, and in manufacturing interests. This trend toward increased competition in labor and small business enterprises caused conflict, generated racial hostilities, and led to antinarcotics legislation.

Coming from another culture, speaking a different language, and being unskilled, the Chinese moved to ghettos where they could find fellowship, information on available work, and a buffer from the dominant white society. As the Chinese population grew, Chinatown became politically organized, with persons from different clans uniting into a *hui kuan*, which became confederated into the political arm of the Chinese sector of the city. That is, the Chinese would settle in those parts of Chinatown dominated by persons from similar villages or provinces in China. These *hui kuan* groups would form a political confederation, which made decisions that affected all of the members of Chinatown. This process made Chinatown a very distinctive, stable, and well-organized social entity, and one very visible to the dominant white society.

Another factor that set the Chinese off from the dominant white society was the scarcity of women. "During the entire period of unrestricted immigration (1850E1882) a total of only 8,848 Chinese women journeyed to American shores. In that same period over 100,000 men arrived in the United States."[31] Many of these women could not stand the rigors of frontier life and either died or returned to China, significantly diminishing their number. Generally, the men who came to the United States could not afford to bring their wives and were able to come themselves only because of the credit ticket system. (A system in which a person in this country would loan the traveler the fair which would be repaid by the traveler's labor in this country.) This predominance of men and the inaccessibility of most white women motivated Chinese males to look for recreation in gambling, prostitution, and drugs.

These vices were usually controlled by the *tongs*, or secret societies, organizations that brought in slave girls from the Orient by telling peasant girls that a husband and a new life awaited them in America. The *tongs* had connections with major British opium traders and brought the drugs and the women to West Coast port cities. They also controlled organized gambling, which gained these secret societies a considerable portion of the money that the Chinese laborers had procured in the mines and urban sweatshops of the West. Prostitution, gambling, and the smoking of opium became organized activities in Chinatown, feeding on the needs and deprivations of the lonely, uncared-for Chinese laborers.

At first, the Chinese were just a curiosity to the settlers in the West, but as their numbers grew and they became more visible in their urban ghettos, class tensions began to mount. A negative definition of the Chinese immigrant began to develop. He was described as a "person [who] does not smell very sweetly; his penuriousness; his lying, knavery, and natural cowardice are proverbial; he dwells apart from white persons, herding only with country-men.... They are nicknamed, cuffed about and treated very unceremoniously by every other class."[32] This stereotype became accentuated with references to the immorality of the Chinese and their fondness for gambling, prostitutes, and drugs. The opium dens in which these vices could be purchased became the object of journalistic exposés and the public fear of the "yellow peril."

These dens of illicit pleasure were described as dark, smoke-filled rooms with several areas in which the individual, having purchased opium from the proprietor, could lay down for several hours, or even days, of rapturous enjoyment of the drug. As the Chinese population increased, these dens and the importation of the drug increased proportionately. The most fearful aspect of this process to the dominant white society was the spread of the Chinese and their "morbid delight" eastward. One observer wrote in 1882:

It was soon found that smokers coming East were constantly making converts, so that in a few months' time small and large towns like Truckee, Carson, Reno and many others, each had their smoking dens and their regular customers. Each new convert seemed to take a morbid delight in converting others, and thus the standing army was daily swelled by recruits.[33]

The fear of contagion, rather than the actual act of drug use, seemed to be at the center of the social meaning of drug use, at least for those who manipulated the organs of social power: media and government.

With the first anti-opium legislation being passed in San Francisco (1875), the trend began to move toward the east, with Virginia City, Nevada, passing a similar ordinance the next year, and onward toward the major cities in the Northeast. As the Chinese migrated eastward looking for work, newspaper accounts of "drug sodden, sex-crazed dope fiends that fascinated and horrified the public" followed them.[34] These images motivated those who wielded power within the states and in the various towns to turn to legal sanctions to regulate this social peril. As these local attempts to prohibit opium "became more rigid, sporadic illicit traffic in the drugs began to develop and the effects of one state to eliminate the problem were nullified, it was claimed, by smuggling from near by states where anti-narcotics laws as yet had not been enacted."[35] This caused states with antinarcotics laws to pressure other states to pass similar laws and collectively to pressure the federal government to pass nation-wide ordinances. This pressure to pass laws governing opium found considerable support from those in the South who feared black cocaine users.

The Rise of Segregation Laws and the "Black Cocaine Fiend"

As with Chinese opium smoking, southern blacks became a target for class conflict, and drug use became one point of tension in this larger sociopolitical struggle. During the late nineteenth century, the South was tightening its grip on blacks through state and local laws instituting residential segregation, segregation on public transportation, and reduction in black access to political and economic resources. The turn of the century witnessed the rise of Jim Crow legislation in most of the South:

The mushroom growth of discriminatory and segregation laws during the first two decades of this century piled up a huge bulk of legislation.... Up and down avenues and byways of Southern life appeared with increasing profusion the little signs: "Whites Only" or "Colored"... over entrances and exits, at theaters and boarding houses, toilets and water fountains, waiting rooms and ticket windows.... In many crafts and trades the written or unwritten policies of Jim Crow unionism made segregation superfluous by excluding Negroes from employment.... [Another method of segregation] designated blocks throughout [a] city black or white according to the majority of the residents and forbade any person to live in any block "where the majority of residents on such streets are occupied by those [of a different race]. ... Smaller towns sometimes excluded Negro residents completely.[36]

In addition to residential and occupational segregation, Jim Crow laws also effectively segregated southern blacks from the political process:

[In order to qualify to vote] the Negroes [had to]... learn to read, or acquire sufficient property, and remember to pay the poll tax and to keep the receipt on file, [but] they could even then be tripped by the final hurdle devised for them—the white primary.... [This hurdle was created by] state laws excluding the minority race from participation and converting the primary into a white man's club.[37]

These laws were enforced by a combination of local and state law officials and various self-appointed groups, such as the Ku Klux Klan. To bolster this systematic oppression of blacks in the rural South, local officials and newspapers ran stories on the "black cocaine fiend" and claimed that the drug would make black men insane, vicious, and sexually aroused. Many whites believed that cocaine not only made black men more prone to crime but more "efficient as criminals. Beyond this point it brings on a state of fear or paranoia, during which time the [cocaine] addict might murder."[38] It was thought that cocaine increased the blacks' physical and sexual power, making them sex-crazed and wanton rapists. The fear of blacks raping white women became an increasing part of the white rhetoric against blacks. White racist officials and newspapers professed the need to take all necessary steps to protect white women against the "over-sexed black man." The thirty-two-caliber bullets used by southern police departments were thought to be ineffective against this menace, and many departments were reported to have switched to thirty-eight-caliber revolvers.

Reports began to filter northward to the various professional committees investigating drug use in the United States. The American Pharmaceutical Association indicated in 1901 that "the use of cocaine ... by negroes in certain parts of the country, is simply appalling.... The police officers of these questionable districts tell us that the habitues are made madly wild by cocaine, which they have no difficulty at all in buying, sometimes being peddled around from door to door."[39]

Newspaper reports of black cocaine fiends also abounded in northern newspapers. The chief of police of Washington, D.C., wrote in 1908 that "the cocaine habit is by far the greater menace to society because the victims are generally vicious. The use of this drug superinduces jealousy and predisposes to commit criminal acts."[40] In 1914, the *New York Times* reported that a "young man, who has not been identified, went insane from cocaine poisoning in Battery Park last evening and ran about like a madman. He seized several women who were taking the air on the benches and soon the park resounded with their screams."[41] As with the case of opium, these reports created a growing fear that cocaine would creep into and contaminate the more respectable sectors of society.

In spite of these reports, there were numerous indications that cocaine abuse by blacks was not very common in the South or in any other part of this country at that time. The Georgia State Asylum, for example, studied the admissions record of over 2,100 consecutive black patients over a five-year period and found that there were only "two cocaine users—and these incidental to the admitting diagnosis... hospitalized between 1909 and 1914."[42] Similar findings emerged from a study about this time, conducted in New York's Bellevue Hospital, showing that cocaine addiction among black patients was far below that of any other group.

The evidence indicating a lack of cocaine addiction among blacks is significant and supports the notion that the "black cocaine fiend" scare was more of a political ploy to legitimize southern segregationist policies. It is likely, however, that some blacks, like members of other classes, did use cocaine for medical purposes. Blacks, especially poor rural ones, were especially prone to disease. Their mortality rates for pneumonia, tuberculosis, pulmonary hemorrhage, gastroenteritis, and typhoid were from two to six times higher than those of whites. This, coupled with their relatively low income and their inaccessibility to good medical facilities, made the patent medicine industry a natural source of relief from the pain of these ailments. Unlike their white counterparts, who could enjoy the moral protection of having their drugs prescribed by a physician, the economic status of blacks left their drug use open to outside interpretation. As racial tension increased during the last half of the nineteenth-century, drug use, even when the motive of medicinal relief may have been its root cause, became contaminated with class tensions and hostilities. There is little doubt that the myth of the black cocaine fiend was a product of white fear rather than a reflection of actual cocaine use among southern blacks.

Mexicans, Moral Tensions, and Marijuana Laws

Unlike the opiates and cocaine, which were used by members of both minorities and middle classes, marijuana was used primarily by Mexican-American inhabitants of the Southwest. Because of the lower-class nature of marijuana use, state and local officials were suspicious of the drug as it migrated into this country during the first third of this century. The drug came into the United States by two different routes. The first was from Mexico into Texas, California, and later Colorado with the influx of migrant farm workers and pickers. With this immigration came increased reports by local authorities of the vagrancy, immorality, and violence of these groups, conditions that soon became associated with the use of marijuana. One police captain from the Southwest reported:

I have had almost daily experience with the users of [marijuana] for the reason that when they are addicted to the use they become very violent, especially when they become angry and will attack an officer even if a gun is drawn on him, they seem to have no fear. I have also noted that when under the influence of this weed they have abnormal strength and that it will take several men to handle one man where under ordinary circumstances one man could handle him with ease.[43]

From these and other reports by local newspapers, local officials, and various other investigators, there arose the notion of the violent and extremely strong drug maniac, a dope fiend who is insensitive to pain or the normal means of social control.

The second common route of marijuana into this country was from the West Indies into the port cities along the Gulf of Mexico, especially into New Orleans. Like the marijuana from Mexico, this was imported by the lower classes, usually black seamen from fruit and fishing boats. In the mid-1920s the prevalence of marijuana became a major point of tension for New Orleans legal and health officials. The commissioner of public safety of New Orleans, Dr. Frank Gomila, stated that the importation and distribution of the drug was extremely well organized and amounted to thousands of kilograms a year. More importantly, the newspapers began sensationalizing reports of teenagers smoking "mootas," a nickname for marijuana. The *New Orleans Morning Star* wrote a series on the "marijuana menace" and quoted the New Orleans superintendent of the Children's Bureau as saying that many troublesome children were known to smoke marijuana. Further, he claimed that at least two children had run away because they could not get their "muggles" (another nickname for marijuana).

With the economic boom in the major cities of the Northeast (Chicago, New York, Boston), many individuals of Latin descent from the Southwest and Caribbean areas began to move into these urban areas. Chicago seems to have been the most heavily emigrated by people of Mexican descent, and the result was increasing tension between previously established ethnic groups—especially Polish and Italian—and the newly arriving Mexicans. The police, who were predominantly Irish, along with other ethnic groups, found Mexican customs threatening and an object for considerable police repression. By 1930, the Mexican population of Chicago had reached 30,000, and the other industrial cities on the southern shores of the Great Lakes— Gary, Cleveland, and Detroit—also had considerable numbers of Mexican immigrants. As in New Orleans, the. metropolitan newspapers began to run stories on "muggle smoking" among teenagers. The *Chicago Tribune* lobbied heavily for antimarijuana legislation. An article appeared in 1929 noting that "the number of addicts is growing alarmingly according to authorities, because of the ease with which [marijuana] can be obtained. The habit was introduced a dozen years ago or so by Mexican laborers... but it has become widespread among American youth... even among school children."[44] Although there is considerable evidence that this notion of a marijuana epidemic was vastly overplayed by the media, there are indications that the fundamental tensions between whites and Mexicans that gave rise to this scare were well founded.

A number of prominent researchers at this time indicated considerable police oppression of the Mexican community. "The Mexicans get little protection in the courts. The Mexicans are now learning that you must buy justice. The police searched the Mexican houses without warrants [during the Mexican-Polish troubles] and let the crowd hit their Mexican prisoners while they were in custody."[45] Because of these tensions, many people, not the least of which were police, tended to stereotype Mexicans as hot-blooded, overly emotional, and prone to release their anger in acts of violence and crime. Mexican customs tended to aggravate this stereotype, especially the tendency for Mexicans to carry knives. For Mexicans with a rural peasant and migratory farm-working background, the knife was a normal and useful tool. However, the wearing of a knife in an urban center was taken as a concealed weapon and therefore a symbol of the Mexican's basic nature. It was a small step from this stereotype to the assumption that marijuana facilitated this proclivity toward violence.

As stories sprang up throughout the West, practically every state west of the Mississippi River passed antimarijuana legislation between 1915 and 1933. As in the case of Chinese opium use, the legislation coincided with significant social changes that aggravated class tensions between the ethnic minority (Mexican) and the dominant white interests. Specifically, "Mexican immigration during the first third of the twentieth century increased enormously; the Bureau of Immigration records the entry of 590, 765 Mexicans from 1915 to 1930."[46] With this influx came the rural peasant custom of marijuana use, and, as it began to appear in the larger cities, city officials increased their pressure on local communities and state governments for stricter drug legislation. The newspaper stories in New Orleans, Chicago, and New York added to the general pressure from the less urbanized areas of the Southwest. These and other pressures led to the passage of numerous local and state laws, culminating with the Federal Marijuana Tax Act in 1937. From the time that marijuana was first brought into this country, around 1910, until the passage of this act, a number of local and state laws had prohibited the use of marijuana for nonmedical purposes. However, this federal act and the subsequent uniform state codes regulating marijuana succeeded in insuring that it would not spread beyond the lower classes. From the late 1930s until the late 1960s, the use of marijuana was confined to the lower classes, predominantly urban blacks, Mexicans, and Puerto Ricans.

The differences between the social context of the medical definition of drug use and that of minority drug use are marked. Whereas the medical context supported the ideal of the reduction of pain and the moral integrity of the user, the lower-class user was depicted as pleasure seeking, oversexed, and prone toward violence. The common fear among whites of an expanding and economically threatening minority facilitated the infusion of the "dope fiend" stereotype with all of the emotions felt by the middle classes. There is little doubt of a close association among economic tensions, racial oppression, and the dominance of the negative definition of drug use. However, a closer look at three theoretical perspectives is necessary for there to be an elucidation of how these factors were historically and structurally interrelated in the rise of antidrug legislation

THEORIES, SOCIETY, AND INDIVIDUALS: THE APPLICATION OF SOCIOLOGICAL THEORY TO THE SOCIAL CONTEXT SURROUNDING THE RISE OF ANTIDRUG LEGISLATION

Until the last couple of decades, the discipline of sociology has been dominated by the functionalist perspective. However, the general turmoil of the late 1960s and the early 1970s, at the national and international levels forced sociologists to reconsider their previous acceptance of the functionalist approach in the light of this ubiquitous social conflict. In response, many sociologists turned to previously ignored perspectives that emphasized social conflict as well as the more phenomenologically oriented theories. Although the functionalist, or value consensus, perspective is no longer the only theoretical stance in the limelight of the discipline, it is still of significant merit to require a close scrutiny in terms of the rise of drug laws.

Value consensus, or functionalist, thought assumes that the law is a reflection of the dominant values and sentiments of a society, and the enforcement of these legal standards demonstrates the normative boundaries that define the social order.[47] Durkheim, the classic theorist of this position, termed the "totality of beliefs and sentiments common to the average citizen" as the "collective conscience."[48] This collective set of sentiments was understood to have an existence beyond the will of individuals and acted to constrain antisocial behavior, and hence, produced "order, harmony, and social solidarity."[49]

Durkheim identified two fundamental types of collective conscience, which he visualized as existing on an evolutionary continuum. At the more primitive end of the continuum are small tribes and agrarian villages in which penal or criminal law is the most dominant. The members of these societies react in a "mechanical" manner to deviant behavior; enforcement of the norms is immediate, harsh, and universally supported by the society. However, with industrialization and concomitant occupational division of labor, this homogeneous form of social solidarity is undermined, and then new "organic" forms of solidarity are created. This organic solidarity reflects an increased structural interdependence between newly formed occupational and social groups. When an increasingly diverse social order can no longer depend solely on a homogeneous set of beliefs and sentiments, a more complex instrument is needed to rectify possible strain between divergent groups. This instrument is the state, which no longer reflects a simple mechanical response to deviance in the form of penal law but rather functions to restitute social imbalances by generating a legal structure that ensures both integration of divergent social segments and a stable equilibrium between these units. Hence, from the value consensus perspective, the rise of antidrug legislation from about 1900 to about the 1930s should reflect (1) a fundamental consensus within the social order concerning the proper normative boundaries for controlling drug use, (2) a shift from penal to restitutive forms of sanctioning when handling deviant forms of drug use, and (3) a tendency toward equilibrium between the dominant society and those who are involved in drug abuse. Unfortunately, neither the existential descriptions of drug use nor the historical contexts in which antidrug legislation was implemented support these theoretical propositions.

There was considerable disparity, both within the middle class and between this class and lower-class drug users, concerning the appropriate social meaning for drug use. Although most members of the middle class found an element of social legitimacy in their use of drugs within the medical context, there was considerable ambivalence on the part of users, physicians, and the larger society concerning the problematic effects of these substances. Rather than a fundamental consensus on the value of these drugs, there were men of letters who described the extreme variations drugs had on the human consciousness. Eminent physicians, such as Freud, were well aware of the positive anesthetizing effects of drugs, as well as the generally soporific effect of opium on the addicted user and the paranoid reaction of the cocaine abuser. William Halsted's experiences with both morphine and cocaine, coupled with his ability to maintain a brilliant medical career, reflects the problematic nature of drug use. Halsted shifted in his later life from cocaine to morphine, a drug that had been reputed to induce lethargy in its user, but he did not experience any major shift in his behavior from what it was under the stimulant cocaine. The most extensive existential descriptions of drug use do not reflect the suggested value consensus needed to support the functionalist view.

When viewing the numerically most dominant segments of the middle class who used drugs, women using morphine within the medical context, again this period reflected a lack of clear consensus within this group. What started as a medically supervised system of drug use often evolved into a normless situation in which the patient would gain control over the amount and frequency of the injections. Addiction in this form was widespread and at times infected infants who nursed from the addict. In spite of the negative information available on the effects of drugs, the over-the-counter pharmaceutical trade incorporated both opium and cocaine into its medicines, syrups, and colas. Users, physicians, and pharmacists all varied on the proper social meaning to impute to drug use. Rather than value consensus among the middle class, there was considerable ambiguity and conflict surrounding the reality of drug use.

At the other end of the social scale, members of the lower classes used drugs to escape from the realities of harsh, exploitive labor, to induce personal feelings of pleasure, and, in some cases, for medicinal purposes. Although there is a lack of literature reflecting vivid personal experiences of the part of lower-class users during this time, there is every reason to suspect that their reactions were as problematic as were those of the middle classes. However, even if there was a consensus on the meaning of drug use within this class, there certainly was not one between this class and those who wielded power within the society as a whole. Where the middle class protected itself, at least initially, with the medical definition of drug use, law enforcement, mass media, and political figures characterized lower-class drug use as leading to insanity, violence, and even murder. The meaning of drug use became so entangled with class tensions that a national value consensus was certainly not apparent. Not only was there evidence of a lack of consensus on this issue, but there is some theoretical concern whether the notion of a national consensus is useful in any wider context. "To speak of 'norms of society' is a vast abstraction when we refer to the complex of divergent classes, ethnic groups, cultures, and regions that are part of the United States.... Rather than the unanimity which Durkheim thought essential, norms of tolerance appear functionally necessary to modern society."[50] However, as Gusfield mentioned, constraint and oppression, rather than tolerance, were reflected in the laws relating to drug use for most of the twentieth century. Further, this oppression did not reflect a consensus held by the society; rather it reflected the ideals of a relatively small percentage of the middle class—a percentage, however, who had access to the means for making their views dominate.

Second, value consensus theory suggests that the laws governing drug use would move from penal to restitutive and that considerable effort would be made to integrate members of the deviant subculture into the social order. However, whether penal or restitutive sanctions were imposed on drug users had more to do with the class background of the user than any general evolution of the social order. The first antidrug laws were passed in the West, specifically San Francisco and Virginia City, in 1875. These laws were penal in nature and were designed to oppress, not integrate, drug users (the Chinese) into the dominant social order. This penal approach to drug control has been the dominant form of legislation throughout most of this century. After the first antinarcotics legislation in the West, the federal government attempted to generate its own ordinances and motivate other states to create penal sanctions of their own. This federal legislation came in the form of the Harrison Act (1914), which banned the use of both opiates and cocaine for nonmedicinal use. Twenty-two years later (1936), the federal government extended its legal dominion over the use of marijuana and pressured the individual states to follow suit. Finally, during the 1950s, the government again claimed a massive increase in drug abuse and was influential in increasing the penalties associated with the laws for controlling drug abuse. During each of these twenty-year cycles, the government was not interested in restituting divergent subcultures; rather, it used its extensive influence and coercive powers to impose penal sanctions on those who had a divergent orientation toward drug use.

Only since the early 1970s has there been any attempt to shift toward a restitutive approach. Many state courts have instituted diversion programs in which persons arrested for possession of small amounts of drugs are diverted out of the criminal justice system into a more informal process of case resolution. In most instances, judicial boards review each case and generate less punitive solutions, such as light probation, working in a rehabilitation center, or controlled supervision by the family. This shift in the law has been a reflection not of the evolution of a general American collective conscience but rather of a shift in the composition of those who use drugs.

Third, value consensus theory would indicate a general trend toward a stable equilibrium in law enforcement concerning drug use.

To the contrary, however, the last century of legal control of drug use reflects cycles of disequilibrium, a disequilibrium fostered by the law enforcement agencies themselves. Rather than organs concerned with alleviating tensions and intergroup conflict, and hence generating social equilibrium, law enforcement and mass media groups were instrumental in generating public hysteria against those who used drugs. Thus the state is more easily understood as an instrument of certain dominant groups who wish to solidify their values over less fortunate subcultures rather than a complex social organ that mediates and mitigates intergroup tensions in an increasingly differentiated society.

Finally, unlike the functionalists, the existential-conflict theorist sees the lived experiences and the social meanings these experiences have for the individual members of a society as the cornerstone of sociological research. Hence, one must "study the situational usages first, [and then] try to determine those general dimensions of meaning shared . . . by members in situations felt to be 'moral'; in this way [one] arrives at an abstract analysis of the meanings of moral rules."[51] Here Douglas suggests that a detailed examination of the day-to-day empirical features of a social situation must be addressed prior to the "abstract analysis of the meanings of moral rules." It is from this common point of departure that a clear appreciation of the existential reality of social conflict and drug laws can be obtained and the relevance of sociological theory determined.

THE MORAL ENTREPRENEUR: LABORIOUS LABELLER OR A COOLIE OF CLASS CONFLICT?

An analysis of this topic must focus on more than those who became the subject of antidrug legislation; equally important is the existential conflict surrounding those individuals who created the law. It has been suggested that "rules are the product of someone's initiative . . . the crusading reformer [who] is interested in the content of the rules. The existing rules do not satisfy him because there is some evil which profoundly disturbs him."[52] These individuals purposefully focus on specific social sentiments, arouse these feelings, and use the resulting social momentum against certain behavior that they personally find reprehensible. These moral entrepreneurs arise by virtue of their personal initiative, access to political decision makers, and skillful use of publicity.

In the case of antinarcotics legislation, there were two predominant moral entrepreneurs, during the first half of this century, Hamilton Wright and Harry Anslinger. Hamilton Wright was instrumental in the creation and coordination of several international conferences on drug control, conferences that were crucial to the creation of the emotional climate that generated both international and national legislation. Collins suggests that this ability to manipulate "the means of emotional production" is a key feature in the process of using social conflict as a foundation for the manipulation of a feedback loop that allows one sector of a social order to dominate over other sectors. Through the manipulation of the conferences that developed the "facts" concerning drug use, as well as much of the media coverage of these events, Wright was able to orchestrate a public response that assured the passage of the laws he desired. With the passage of these antinarcotic laws, an enforcement agency, the Federal Bureau of Narcotics, was created to insure compliance. The original head of this agency was Harry Anslinger, a moral entrepreneur in his own right. Anslinger, like Wright before him, used his political position to generate evidence concerning the problem of the "dope fiend," coordinate this evidence into a mass media image, and use this image to generate feelings of "solidarity, fear . . . and a sense of purpose" which Collins suggested was crucial to such a campaign.[53] Where Wright laid the political groundwork in his campaign against opium and cocaine in 1914, Anslinger followed suit twenty years later with his drive against the use of marijuana.

Any theory that claims to explain the rise of drug laws must address all of the major contextual aspects of the social values that conflicted over the issue. It must explain not only the values and strategies of those who generated the laws but also the structural tensions that surrounded their work. As Collins points out:

A society is an aggregate of individuals, is not integrated; common values do not operate to hold them all together. . . . What we call a society is nothing more than a shifting network of groups and organizations, held together by one or both of these principles—coalition of interests, or dominance and submission.[54]

In this case there was a strong coalition between the middle class and the moral entrepreneur, which resulted in domination over the values and life-styles of the lower-class drug users.

The key value surrounding the drug controversy was the issue of one's personal will and the effect a drug might have on it. Members of the middle class tended to react with fear and anxiety to the specter of a weak will and the social malaise that might result. However, because of the medical context of their drug use, they were not considered to be immoral, although the loss of will was a source of considerable personal consternation. Hence, the members of the middle class tended to value a strong will but were not socially degraded because they were not seen as having intended for this effect to have resulted from their drug use.

A close look at the core middle-class value of a strong will suggests three interrelated features: the user making the decision to use drugs independent of outside coercion, a clear understanding of the effects of the drug, and a desire to remain free of any debilitating effects. The medical context met these fundamental tenets. The physician-patient information loop was premised on a trust relationship, not coercion by the physician. The assumption of adequate professional knowledge on the part of the physician assured the patient that a medicinal effect would result from the drug. Finally, there was no conscious intent on the part of the user to become addicted to the drug. The problem of addiction, with this set of values, was primarily an issue of moderating the dosage rather than an issue of social or moral pathology.

These three features of the core value of a free will were inverted for lower-class drug users. Their drug use was seen to be a product of social coercion in which an individual, through pressure within the social class, would take up cigarette smoking, then alcohol, and ultimately drugs. As these coercive social influences expanded, they would ultimately threaten, and possibly engulf, members of the middle class. In a similar manner, whereas middle-class users were perceived as unaware of the negative effects of the drug, lower-class users were understood not only to be aware of these effects but took the drug specifically for these effects. Hence, the lower-class users not only willfully desired the lascivious effects of these drugs but consciously became caught up in their effects. Not only was the primary use of one's personal will misdirected, but the individual consciously desired the very destruction of that valued psychological faculty.

When the interplay between middle- and lower-class drug use is taken within the larger historical context of the turn of the century, the rise of antidrug legislation was not simply the imposing of middle-class values on the lower classes, as portrayed by the labelling theorists. Rather, there were conflicts between these two groups in terms of the ways in which they related to the core value of one's will. Historical accounts do indicate that members of the lower classes took drugs for different reasons than did members of the middle classes. The antidrug laws were not the reflection of the whim of several politically powerful, but morally misguided, individuals. Rather the moral entrepreneur was situated at the heart of conflicting groups with different life experiences, different perceptions of morality, and divergent access to political levers of control. Variations of the intentions to use drugs were simply a reflection of deeper schisms of class conflict.

Labelling theorists tended to take an extreme position in reaction to the functionalist's assertion of an absolute value consensus and assumed that there were no commonly held core values within a major portion of the social order. Any indication of universal values, they argued, was the product of the moral entrepreneur. As Warren and Johnson note, "Although evidence indicates the use and upholding of some 'core values' in everyday life of members of a society, labelling theorists have refused to investigate, or acknowledge their plausibility."[55] Hence, the work of the labelling theorists gives useful insights into the values and experiences of those who were instrumental in creating these antidrug laws, but they ignore both the existential existence of core values held by those who are affected by these laws, as well as the complex structural interplay of values, power, and manipulation that existed among various groups that shaped this legislation.

Class Conflict, International Conferences, and Legislative Clout

The flow of emotions through the social context that surrounds the rise of drug laws has been well documented. Gusfield's assertion that the law can reflect the conflict over fundamental class values, the symbolic domination of one class over another, and the coordination of the emotions emanating from large-scale social tensions has been developed in terms of the rise of drug laws. What is of concern now is the existential question of the strategies and tactics used by moral entrepreneurs to coordinate their crusade. Collins, taking a general theoretical position, suggests that those who wish to control "the means of emotional production . . . [must use the] ecological conditions that bring individuals together for emotional encounters, control the resources for putting on an emotional display and coordinate the resources to mobilize accumulated techniques for emotional manipulation."[56] Each of these three aspects of the means for emotional production was used, in varying degrees, by both Hamilton Wright and Harry Anslinger.

The two decades that preceded the passage of the Harrison Act witnessed a significant expansion of the U.S. political boundaries, which created a new ecological environment that had to be tamed by the federal administration. Prior to 1900, the United States was ecologically bound by oceans to the west and east and two, somewhat stable but weaker, powers to the north and south. However, the continued drive to expand westward resulted in the Spanish-American War of 1898, in which the United States defeated the decaying feudal empire of Spain and acquired the Philippines, Guam, Puerto Rico, and Cuba. With the expansion of the nation-state into the new environment of the Pacific, coupled with the lure of extensive Chinese markets, American political and economic interests were eager to create new social structures for control and domination. Secretary of State John Hay, proclaimed an "open door" policy, in which the United States would enjoy an increased footing in all eastern markets and significant access to all of the ports over which the European nations had previously held hegemony.

As the United States inherited new economic markets and a more significant international stature, it also faced a drug problem. Opium had been shipped by the British from the Middle East and India to China for over a century. Although there was some moral outcry from sectors of the British population from time to time, the trade continued because of its lucrative tax revenue for the British colonial system. Further, British shipping interests were well aware that their withdrawal from the market would not seriously curtail the importation of opium to China and the Far East Pacific area. Other nations that had played a minor role at the time—German, French, and some U.S. merchants—would simply increase their operations, and the Chinese themselves would become adept at growing the opium poppy. Although opium trade was of questionable moral status, the realities of the market would determine economic policy.

Because of this, the American colonial administration of the Philippines faced an opium problem in their newly acquired islands. The Chinese had continued the British tradition by importing opium into the Philippines for more than a century. During this period, the use of opium among the Chinese minority had become well established and had spread to a significant part of the Philippine population. The Spanish colonial government had attempted to control the use of opium by creating a government monopoly on the importation, sales, and medical use of the drug. To import and distribute the drug, the government contracted merchants who then had to pay a tax and agree to sell only to the Chinese minority. However, when the Americans won the war and the Spanish control of opium was destroyed, importation and distribution began to increase. This, coupled with the cholera epidemic in 1902, during which opium was used extensively by Filipinos for medical purposes, created a serious problem for the new American administration.

As the ecological boundary that surrounded the nation-state shifted into new and exotic areas of the Pacific and men in important social and political positions began to fear a new moral threat looming from these areas, the stage was set for the entrance of the moral entrepreneur. The Roosevelt administration found such an individual in the personage of Hamilton Wright. Because of his experience with tropical diseases and his personal influence with the existing Washington administration, Wright was able to become the central figure in the creation of the emotional display necessary for the passage of the federal legislation. This took the form of international conferences on drug trade.

Wright was astute in his control of the accumulated techniques of emotional manipulation. With the rise of industrialization and the increased sacredness of scientific knowledge, these accumulated techniques took the form of statistical surveys and estimates of drug abuse from official organizations. In preparation for the conference, to be held in Shanghai, Dr. Wright launched a national survey to collect information on opium use, importation, and distribution in this country. He also requested that other nations, especially the major growers of opium (Persia, Turkey, India, and China) and distributors (England, France, and Germany), gather information on drug production, distribution, and use. Although many persons in government took exception to his frenetic attempts to take complete control of the anti-opium movement, Dr. Wright was convinced that the Americans should lead the way. As is characteristic of moral entrepreneurs, along with his efforts to gain information, he was also prone to exaggerate the horrors resulting from the lack of control of opium. In a letter to the Episcopal bishop of the Philippines, he indicated that "an enormous amount of opium and its derivates and cocaine was supplied to the army and navy, but that he had been assured that the drugs had been stolen by unscrupulous persons in the medical department and sold surreptitiously in our larger cities."[57] Whether this was true was never satisfactorily proven, but it did buttress Wright's moral crusade against the drug.

If Wright was to bring together an international conference in order to create an emotional display in favor of drug control, it was imperative that America have exemplary opium laws as a model for the rest of the world. But the "United States had no national laws limiting or prohibiting importation, use, sale, or manufacture of opium . . . and derivatives."[58] Thus because the conference was to be held in Shanghai within a couple of months, there was an obvious need for quick national legislation. In December 1909, the U.S. Congress responded with the needed legislation: a statute prohibiting the importation of opium used for smoking into the Philippines and the United States. This law, however, was of little practical significance because there was no mention of controlling opiates administered by physicians (the major source of morphine addiction), and no specialized law enforcement agency designed to enforce the law, essentially a duplication of a Food and Drug Administration law already on the books. Indeed the head of the enforcement of the Pure Food and Drug Act of 1906 pointed out that section II of the existing act provided for the banning of any imported drug that was detrimental to the health of the people of the United States.[59] Nevertheless the law functioned as a display of congressional feelings concerning the problem of drug abuse, a display that Wright used to bolster his desire for international control, in spite of the indication that the law had little practical merit in keeping drug smuggling under control.

Armed with this statute from his home country, Wright set off for the Shanghai Conference to admonish other nations to join the fight against narcotics. At the conference, Wright felt his efforts were successful—a success he attributed to the congressional passage of this law. More specifically, the participating nations at the conference resolved that each nation should initiate a program for the suppression of opium smoking, that each should reexamine its own laws in regard to regulating opiate use for nonmedical purposes, and that no nation could export opium to any other nation whose laws prohibit its importation. But here too the resolution seems to have had more of a display function than a practical legal impact. Of those nations involved in the conference, two of the most significant producers of opium either did not send a delegation (Turkey) or sent a mere merchant as a representative (Persia), so neither was legally, diplomatically, or morally bound to the conference's resolutions. France and Germany, two nations involved in the transportation of opiates, sent representatives but let it be known that they were not especially concerned with the problem. Further, Great Britain and the Netherlands requested that the meeting be only a conference involved in fact finding and empowered only to make recommendations, not internationally binding commitments, which would give them the needed political room to reconstruct their trade relations with India and China in a manner most in line with their economic interests. Finally, there was no mention of an international police organization to enforce any dictates that came from the conference.

Although this conference did not produce practical legal measures for the control of opiates, it did generate emotional momentum at the international level that could be used for the passage of significant legislation at the national level. Given the fact that numerous powerful nations were interested in discussing the problem, even if many lacked the concern to take the issue much further, the conference acted as a symbolic manifestation of international concern over the drug problem. As Gusfield points out, "Symbolic acts [functions] as forms of rhetoric [and] organize the perceptions, attitudes, and feelings of observers."[60] It was this symbolic act that Wright was successful in producing at the conference, and he was intent on using it as a rhetorical base for generating an information loop that would structure public and governmental sentiments on the national level.

Wright's coordination of information between the national and international political domains reflects the way in which seemingly unrelated areas of conflict are often integrated by the politically powerful and used for their own ends. As Collins points out, "These techniques [of emotional manipulation] are resources to be used in other conflicts, and the control of these means is itself ... the result of other forms of conflict."[61] Within the context of antidrug legislation, this would suggest that the initially unrelated political conquest of the Pacific became a resource used by the moral entrepreneur in his quest for a national drug law. Wright gained power by being involved in an area (the South Pacific as a physician) that was embroiled in conflict (Spanish-American War) and used this as a basis for his claim of expertise in spearheading an international conference on drug abuse. This, in turn, enabled Wright to have a significant amount of control over the means of emotional manipulation (gathering of scientific data) "which would be used in other conflicts"—in this case, the conquest of the cocaine problem.

The Cocaine Problem: A White Solution for Black Problems

If the conflict that surrounded America's intervention into the Far East was the stage on which Wright mobilized support for the control of the opium trade, racial conflict in the South became the resource for generating concern for control of cocaine. Although Wright himself was probably concerned with controlling cocaine and was not a racist, his antinarcotics crusade served to focus attention on black cocaine users.

Since Congress had passed an antiopium smoking act just prior to the Shanghai Conference, Wright shifted his attention to cocaine and claimed that its effects were more appalling than any other drug. In a report to Congress, Wright suggested that "the use of cocaine by the negroes of the South is one of the most elusive and troublesome questions which confront the enforcement of the law in most of the Southern States.... The Drug is commonly sold in whiskey dives, and ... the combination of low-grade spirits and cocaine makes a maddening compound."[62] As with all of the repressive laws established in the South after the end of Reconstruction in 1877, laws against cocaine would be effective in keeping blacks "in their place." Wright saw that he would need the support of southern Democratic congressmen to get a more stringent antinarcotics law passed by Congress. By appealing to southerners' fear of the black cocaine fiend, Wright was able to overcome their fear of increased federal police powers inherent in the passage of any federal legislation. Ultimately, southerners were more afraid of blacks than of increased federal power to regulate these drugs.

Evidence suggests that this too was an elaborate staging device in which the moral entrepreneur uses social conflict as a resource for coordinating the creation of an information system. The statistical breakdown of cocaine users in the South at that time indicated that drug psychosis (the medical term for "drug fiend") was much more common among whites than blacks. Although the statistical gathering process at that time was not impervious to error, only 3 blacks were found to be suffering from cocaine-related psychosis during a five-year period in Georgia, while 142 whites were so diagnosed.[63] These and other supporting studies reflected the lack of accurate information in many of Wright's statements. However, he seems to have been more interested in "organizing perceptions, attitudes, and feelings" than in attending to the social basis he claimed to be portraying.

With increases in domestic concern over both opium and cocaine, Wright returned to the international forum to stage further displays of the need for stricter drug control. Again, he coordinated efforts between an international conference and national attempts to generate antidrug legislation—the former being held at the Hague in 1912 and the latter being manifested in the Foster bill of 1911. As was the case with congressional legislation just prior to the Shanghai Conference, Wright, with the backing of the State Department, pressured Congress to pass more stringent legislation to insure America's symbolic status at the Hague Convention. This time he pressed to expand legislation beyond opium used for smoking to all nonmedical use of opiates, cocaine, and other habit-forming drugs. Although Wright was less than pleased with the ultimate outcome of either the Foster bill (which was defeated) or the Hague Convention, he was able to gain some international support for the inclusion of cocaine on this list of controlled drugs.

In spite of the success of including cocaine in the antidrug campaign, Wright was disappointed that these recent efforts did not move significantly beyond the symbolic level to practical control measures. The major problem with the Hague Convention was that it simply duplicated the staging aspects of the previous Shanghai Conference. In Wright's words, the Hague Article "is weak in that the powers only pledge themselves to use their best efforts to control or cause to be controlled those who manufacture, import, sell, distribute, or export morphine, cocaine, and their respective salts."[64] Although no international organization was instituted to control drug traffic, the resolution gave clear support for Wright's efforts to generate such legislation on the domestic level. Two years later when Wright again focused his efforts on coordinating the passage of domestic legislation, he had finally developed the resources necessary for its passage. As Collins suggests, the ability to control the distribution of resources (in this case, legislative power) itself is affected by the distribution of resources resulting from other forms of conflict.

Wright's ability to create an international display of America as the moral vanguard against the evils of international narcotics trade did much to promote the passage of key antinarcotics legislation, the Harrison Act of 1914. This legislation specifically limited the possession, processing, and sale of "opium and coca leaves, and compounds, manufactures, salts, derivatives or preparations thereof" except by persons registered with the federal government.[65] It was designed to "provide ways in which these drugs may be purchased and held in possession by registered persons" to insure their use for medical purposes only.[66] Given constitutional restrictions, the Congress was obligated to pass a law requiring each person engaged in a drug-related transaction (such as buying, selling, dispensing, or prescribing) to register and pay a federal tax, which the government could use to structure a licensing system that would control the flow of drugs into legitimate medical use. The Treasury Department, which was responsible for enforcing tax legislation, was directed to "make needful rules and regulations for carrying out the provisions of this act" and so created the Narcotics Division of the U.S. Treasury.[67]

CONCLUSIONS

The rise of drug laws around the turn of this century are not easily explained by some traditional sociological theories. The functionalist view, although a major contribution to the discipline as a whole, has not been useful in elucidating the complex historical, structural, or individual variables that constitute this issue. This view focuses only on the macrolevel and gives little insight into the particular strategies influential individuals used in generating these laws. Further, the assumption that these laws reflect a social consensus on the issue of moral values, create clear normative boundaries for establishing social equilibrium, and evolve from penal to restitutive sanctions has not been born out. Clearly, the history of antidrug legislation over the last century reflects conflict over social values, disequilibrium, and shifts due to class structure.

A more fruitful theoretical approach is the existential-conflict perspective, which emphasizes an easy movement between the micro and macro perspectives as well as an emphasis on the role of structural tensions, human emotions, and the symbolic aspects of the law. This view accepts the basic findings of the labelling theorist, a perspective that has dominated drug research for more than three decades but consciously moves beyond its limitations. Where the labelling theorists have seen key individuals, the moral entrepreneurs, as the ultimate cause of antidrug legislation, the existential-conflict theorists locate these individuals within the larger structural and historical context. By integrating the specifics of the labelling research with the larger structural trends, a clear, concise, and comprehensive view of this issue is possible.

The primary structural tension around 1900 was between the white middle class and three expanding minorities—the Chinese in the West, blacks in the South, and Mexicans in the Southwest—each moving from their previous state of isolation (Chinese in western Chinatowns, blacks from slavery, and the Mexicans from the Southwest territories). As each group began to migrate from these racial cloisters toward the rural fields and industrial cities where work was most available, their visibility and willingness to work for less money than whites did created tension. The latter part of the nineteenth century reflected an attempt by the dominant social institutions to reestablish a system of racial isolation relative to these groups. Antidrug legislation was just one aspect of this process.

These structural tensions fed easily into the stereotype of the dope fiend that became the symbol for rallying these negative human emotions. Just as the minorities were seen to lack ambition, self-discipline, and a strong will, the dope fiend was portrayed in a similar manner. Just as the racial minorities were becoming more visible and whites feared that they would eventually infect their respectable classes, the dope fiend was seen as a similar threat. The image of the dope fiend was a simple, emotionally salient, and stable reflection of larger structural and historical tensions.

Generally, middle-class drug use received a positive social definition within the medical context in which it developed. However, the infusion of class and racial tensions into the negative stereotype of lower-class drug users caused this definition of drug use to prevail. Men of letters, such as De Quincey, Blair, and Baudelaire, first described the negative aspects of the drug experience. Although the problematic nature of drug use was also recognized by the more sensitive members of the medical profession, their desire to find simple answers to complex physical problems led the profession to endorse the opiates and later cocaine without understanding the full significance of their effects. Not until the first decade of this century did the profession fully recognize the need for stricter normative controls.

With the declining support of the positive definition of these drugs by the medical profession and the rise of structural tensions between middle and lower classes, the stage was set for the moral entrepreneur. As Collins pointed out, the persons who desire to "control the means of emotional production" must meet a number of strategic criteria. They must use the ecological conditions to bring powerful individuals together for an emotional encounter, control the resources for an emotional display, and mobilize the techniques for emotional manipulation. Hamilton Wright, the organizing power behind the Harrison Act, successfully met each of these criteria. By gathering information from local and state officials who feared minority expansion and had accepted the stereotype of the dope fiend, Wright was able to control the resources for an emotional display. With this solid political foundation, he used the new ecological conditions of the

U.S. presence in the Far East to coordinate a number of international conferences, which gave increased credibility to his facts and stature to the antidrug movement. Acting as a mediating agent for local, state, and international bodies concerned with the drug issue, Wright was able to mobilize the emotions necessary for the passage of the desired legislation.

The existential-conflict theory benefits considerably from the recent labelling theorist's use of the idea of an information feedback loop. By focusing on the role of information control in the creation, circulation, and expansion of these definitions, it is possible to gain a clear conception of the relative significance of all of the factors that affected the rise of drug laws. As the structural tensions between minorities and the dominant white culture increased, these emotions began to feed into the dope fiend stereotype. This infusion of deep, structurally generated emotion into the symbol of the dope fiend created the momentum necessary for the moral entrepreneur to structure the passage of the laws that imposed the label of deviant on drug users. As Gusfield has pointed out, the actual subject of the law, whether it is the drinker or dope fiend, is only a symbolic representation of larger social tensions. With the passage of each new law at the local and state levels, more momentum and legitimation was infused in this stereotype until finally, in 1914, the Harrison Act was passed. With this act, the drug issue shifted from the realm of collective behavior to the problems surrounding the role of bureaucratic organizations and the drug issue. The individual drug user often found the existential reality of drug use problematic, and the social definition of drug use was highly problematic until it became formalized with the passage of federal legislation. So too the organizational issues that surrounded the creation and expansion of the Federal Bureau of Narcotics reflected the existential issues of problematic social definitions, social conflict, and information control.

2 ORGANIZATIONAL THEORY, SOCIAL CONFLICT, AND DRUG LAW ENFORCEMENT

Weber, as well as the more recent conflict theorists, saw modern iety's shift toward large-scale bureaucratic organizations as the most ffective and legitimate means of handling social problems. The drug problem was no exception. With the passage of the Harrison Act, the law enforcement fight against drugs shifted from the more or less ad hoc tactics of Hamilton Wright and his supporters to a more institutional approach of the Federal Bureau of Narcotics (FBN). Now that the fight against drug use could be staged from an institutional base, it was crucial that the momentum developed by Wright's campaign be continued in a manner that both strengthened this institution and increased its scope over the control of drugs.

Weber developed the classic model of the modern bureaucracy with its hierarchical chain of command, formally defined and fixed role obligations, decisions based on technical skills, and impersonal procedures for meeting organizational goals. Like most other bureaus, the FBN fit this general typology in many respects. The hierarchical command was headed by a commissioner who reported directly to the secretary of the treasury. Given the fact that the federal law was a tax initiative, the Treasury Department was responsible for its enforcement. From an organizational perspective, this was efficient because the other two federal agencies that would participate in controlling the smuggling aspect of the drug problem, the U.S. Customs and Coast Guard, were also under the Treasury Department. Ideally this hierarchical structure would be coordinated by objective and impartial procedural guidelines, which would act to define and limit role obligations, determine the technical knowledge

on which decisions would be made, and implement impersonal procedures for meeting the organizations's goals.

Neither Weber nor the modern conflict theorists assumed that
these features would adequately describe all, or even the most important, features of modern organizations, however. The interplay
between this organizational ideal and the existential reality of how a
particular organization actually operates is best described by Collins:
"The 'organization' is only people attempting to get certain things for
themselves and using other people as the means... 'organizational
structure' is only a way of referring to how people behave repetitively
towards each other.''[1] Here Collins is referring to a major existential
tension that exists within organizational structure. On the one hand,
members are required to interact in repetitive ways that ensure the
adherence to standardized procedures and fixed roles; on the other
hand, they are interested in achieving wealth, power, and recognition
for themselves, values that are zero sum (that is, the amount accumulated by one individual is necessarily deprived from some other
individual) and lead to conflict. This tension between organized or
routinized interaction and the desire to maximize one's interest is
inherent at every level of organized life. This conflict within the
organizational structure is often accompanied by feelings of anxiety
and personal conflict. As Douglas suggested, "These conflicts produce greater frustrations... within individuals, so they develop massive 'frontwork' and 'prefigured justifications'... for public presentation to protect their private personal feelings and lives within the
organization.''[2] Hence, although the ideal typification of a bureaucratic organization may exist to some degree, a far more significant
aspect of these structures is the existential conflicts concerning organizational rules, tensions between individuals desiring personal gain,
and the fronts constructed to hide these realities.

Although the interface between bureaucratic ideals and the existential reality of social conflict is often ubiquitous within an organization, there are ways to reduce this disparity. One way is to increase the
scope of administrative jurisdictions, which creates occupational
opportunities for aggressive individuals at all levels of the agency.
Not only does this help satiate the human need for power but also,
especially among the administrative elite, it confers the concomitant
rewards of wealth and status. A key lever for the increase of power

and administrative discretion is the organizational control of legal ambiguities. When the organization can identify, dominate, and encompass an area of legal ambiguity, it can create administrative procedures that act as a foundation for its continued existence. Further, it can claim expertise in this area and control the structuring and dissemination of information on the ambiguous issue. This was one of the basic strategies of the FBN in its early years of growth.

FROM CHARISMATIC TO BUREAUCRATIC POWER: THE ORGANIZATIONAL CONTROL OF LEGAL AMBIGUITIES

Weber initially suggested that charismatic individuals (such as moral entrepreneurs) arise during times of conflict and are instrumental in generating the organizational structure (such as a bureaucracy) necessary for insuring the continuation of their ideals. Collins expands on this notion by integrating an insight from Crozier's *The Bureaucratic Phenomenon* that bureaucratic organizations may substantially increase their power through the organizational control of ambiguous situations. In short, organizational power gravitates to those who are able to handle unexpected situations.

The Harrison Act initially was designed to ensure medical supervision of drug use and implicitly gave physicians considerable professional discretion in determining the proper use of such drugs. However, the wording of the statute was not specific on the exact parameters of medical discretion; it stated only that each person who used the drug must register with the federal government. This could have been easily accomplished by having the physician fill out the federal registration form as part of the patient-physician relationship. Thus both the physician and the government would be meeting the requirements of the law, and reasonable parameters could be placed on the drug problem. However, the FBN used this ambiguity as a crack through which it could thrust its administrative prerogative and develop considerable discretionary power over drugs.

Within a decade after the passage of the Harrison Act, the Treasury Department was able to control this area of ambiguity and develop extremely harsh standards for the control of these drugs. The standards restricted these drugs from those who desired them for nonmedical purposes and also seriously undermined the discretionary power of the medical profession in their use. Specifically, the Treasury Department's decisions limited medical use to those cases in which there was "professional treatment, in the attempted cure of the habit, but... the purpose of providing the user with morphine sufficient to keep him comfortable by maintaining his customary use" was regarded as a violation of the Harrison Act.[3] This organizational attempt to control ambiguous areas of the act continued in another administrative regulation three months later indicating that "a physician acting in accordance with proper medical practice may prescribe or dispense narcotics for the relief of acute pain or for any acute condition... [for] diseases known to be incurable... [but] mere addiction alone is not recognized as an incurable disease."[4]

What initially seemed to be a legislative attempt to restrict the dispensing of drugs to the professional practice of medicine was administratively reconstructed, seriously curtailing doctors' ability to use their professional discretion in the treatment of addicts. Any prescription or treatment that the Narcotics Division did not consider within proper medical practice or was deemed to keep the addict comfortable opened the physician to federal prosecution. This caused many physicians to be reluctant to treat addicts for fear of possible prosecution. If the addict could not legitimately receive drugs, he could either withdraw or turn to illegitimate sources for drugs.

The Supreme Court did not halt this trend. In the first test case, *W. S. Webb* v. *United States* (1919), the Court upheld the government's claim that prescriptions for drugs that provide users with morphine sufficient to keep them comfortable are in violation of the law. After this Court decision, the Treasury Department issued a memorandum to the narcotics enforcement personnel indicating that the Court favored the prosecution of physicians who distribute drugs "to a person popularly known as a 'dope fiend', for the purpose of gratifying his appetite for the drug" as in violation of the Harrison Act.[5] The problem, of course, involved the ambiguity of what cases were attempts to cure a drug addict and which were prescription sufficient to keep such a person comfortable. The courts indicated that each case must stand on its own merits, but the drift of the initial Supreme Court decision was taken as an absolute repudiation of the medical position by the Treasury Department. The Court continued to support the law enforcement position with another decision, *United States* v. *Behrman* (1922), in which it ruled that any prescription by a doctor, in private or public capacity, was in violation of the Harrison Act. This decision formally outlawed clinics and forbade private practitioners treating addicts, which made the law enforcement approach dominant. In drying up all access to drugs by addicts, the government felt that the problem of addiction would be curtailed. By this decision, the past ambiguities inherent in *Webb* concerning proper treatment of addicts, as opposed to prescriptions that kept them comfortable, were irrelevant. By this decision, doctors were deprived of the defense that they had acted in good faith since "Dr. Behrman was convicted despite the fact that the prosecution stipulated that he had prescribed drugs in order to treat and cure addicts."[6] The FBN was not interested in developing complex programs that included a medical approach to the rehabilitation of drug addicts. Rather, they wanted to consolidate their organizational hegemony over the fluid area of ambiguous legislation and conflicting court decisions that characterized this area.

In a later decision, however, the Supreme Court acted more as a mediating agency between the law enforcement and medical approach to drug control. Instead of closing the issue, this later court decision attempted to develop broad guidelines within which a rational and humane drug policy could be developed. At one end were the initial *Webb* and *Behrman* cases, which emphasized a law enforcement approach concerned over the ability of an addict to control his habit and the need for tight constraint on medical dispensing of drugs. On the other was *Lindner* v. *United States* (1925), which explicitly repealed these assumptions and stated that drug addiction is a disease that can best be handled within the physician-patient relationship. The *Linder* decision was important because it represented an alternative interpretation of the Harrison Act that could have been a legitimating basis for a more noncriminal approach to the narcotics problem. Although the *Lindner* decision did not specifically repudiate the doctrines drawn from these previous decisions, it did indicate that these cases involved the flagrant abuse of the physician's discretionary powers and that their conclusions must be seen to emanate from this context. The Court stated:

It [the Harrison Act] says nothing of "addicts" and does not undertake to prescribe methods for their medical treatment. They are diseased and the proper subjects for such treatment, and we cannot possibly conclude that a physician acted improperly or unwisely or for other than medical reasons solely because he has dispensed to one of them... tablets of morphine or cocaine to relieve the conditions of addiction.[7]

The Court specifically addressed the *Webb* and *Behrman* decisions, reiterating that the Harrison Act was initially and essentially a tax measure that "must not be construed as forbidding every prescription for drugs... when designed to alleviate an addict's pain."[8] This decision, and its explicit expansion of organizational discretion toward a medical approach for reducing addiction, could have been the basis of a more humane solution to the drug problem. However, law enforcement agencies paid little or no attention to this later decision and generated policies for the apprehension, adjudication, and sanctioning of addicts in terms of the assumptions implicit in the prior decisions.

Just as with the initial creation of the antidrug legislation, the general strategy of the FBN was to spread and amplify the negative feedback loop. However, instead of just building public sentiment for this negative definition, the bureau administrators were coordinating and contorting the law to meet its organizational desires. With the new-found, although not unanimous, support from the Supreme Court, this feedback loop developed practical enforcement capabilities. Not only would this loop create a symbolic status for the deviant, but it would also now have legal consequences for these individuals. As in the case of its initial development, the definition became infused with motives having little to do with the drug problem. Now bureaucratic aggrandizement added to the momentum of this definition.

The government's intrusion into an area of medical discretionary powers was not popular with the medical profession. Although there was considerable conflict between these two groups, neither was initially organized or entrenched enough to displace the other. The Narcotics Division of the Treasury Department had just been formed and had not yet developed an extensive political or enforcement apparatus to ensure complete compliance with its stated desires. And the medical profession, although distrustful of this new government threat, was not organized enough to counter the momentum of the antinarcotics movement. A compromise was necessary. As Collins suggests, the more equal the power resources and the more comprehensive the surveillance between two groups, the more likely the quest for conciliation and group inclusion.[9]

Physicians had cogently argued that government regulations were too arbitrary to meet the complexities of individual cases of addiction. Addicts had to be treated within the medical context, they held, and a government-supported program of medical clinics could prove to be the best compromise for meeting this problem.

From 1918 until it was abruptly suspended by the federal government in 1922, there was a national program for the clinical treatment of drug addiction. This was an extension of clinics set up by various local, state, and federal agencies for the treatment of tuberculosis, mental illness, and syphilis. Initially, the Treasury Department favored a short-term clinic program to cure those addicts who had inadvertently become dependent on the drug. During this period, clinics sprang up in almost all of the major cities in the United States; the largest were in New York City, New Orleans, Shreveport, Atlanta, New Haven, and Albany. These were sponsored mainly by municipal and state funds but were closely scrutinized by the Treasury Department.

Tensions that stemmed from the conflict between the Treasury Department's law enforcement approach and the medical profession's healing view were reflected in the clinic program. Treasury and local police officials tended to be suspicious of most clinics, believing they were maintaining the addicts' comfort rather than curing them. Law enforcement agencies frequently investigated these clinics, even those that apparently had impeccable programs. Ultimately the New York City clinic became the prime example of an ineffective clinic from the perspective of the law enforcement agencies. This clinic, like many others throughout the country, was overburdened. It had an intake of over 800 addicts per day and 7,464 registered under its care. Ideally, each addict was given a decreasing dose of drugs per day until he showed signs of withdrawal. During this crucial period of withdrawal, the patient was offered a bed at the Riverside Hospital until the cure was complete. However, because of the case load, addicts would often be able to acquire several doses a day by coming to the clinic at different times. Theft of drugs was also a problem and, in some cases, doctors were bribed to provide drugs. Although serious transgressions were the exception, the negative reports by law enforcement officials, coupled with major mass media buildup, gave the clinic program a less than desirable social image. By 1922, the thrust of the law enforcement approach outweighed that of the medical view, and the clinics were closed.

Instead of solving the social problem, this policy simply completed the negative feedback loop by making the addict subject to arrest and legal sanctions. Increases in drug arrests further inflamed public sentiment against the deviant and for the law enforcement administration. Statistics on federal arrests and convictions during the period of clinic operations, (table 1) increased federal law enforcement pressure.[10]

Table 1

FEDERAL ARRESTS AND CONVICTIONS FOR NARCOTICS LAW VIOLATIONS, SELECTED YEARS

Year	Arrests	Convictions
1918	888	392
1919	1,008	582
1920	3,477	908
1921	4,014	1,583
1925	10,297	5,600

Note: The clinics were open from 1918 through 1921. They were closed in 1925.

Arrests and convictions began to increase as the addict became more stigmatized as a criminal by the Treasury Department and the courts. As the open and legitimate avenues for obtaining narcotics closed, addicts became more dependent on underground sources. Thus the legal process directly propagated a new class of criminals by restricting addicts' access to legal drugs.

The Bureau of Narcotics had solidified its control over the discretionary use of drugs, whether that discretion emanated from the medical profession or an individual user. The techniques of emotional displays, played out in the mass media, and key administrative regulations supported by Supreme Court decisions all contributed to this agency's control over organizational ambiguities. As Crozier has pointed out regarding organizational power, "Change will not come gradually.... It will wait until a serious question pertaining to an important dysfunction can be raised.... It will be decided upon at a higher level and applied ... in a way to get rid of local [in this case medical] privileges that have developed around the rules."[11] This explanation adequately describes the basic organizational strategy of the FBN and became its strategy in attacking another drug— marijuana.

THE MORAL ENTREPRENEUR: A LABORIOUS LABELLER OR A MENACE TO MEXICANS?

The labelling theorists, Becker and Lindesmith, saw the FBN, and especially its commissioner, Harry Anslinger, as the major impetus in a two-pronged attack against marijuana. Specifically, "The Bureau's efforts took two forms: cooperating in the development of state legislation affecting the use of marijuana, and providing facts and figures for journalistic accounts."[12] In an approach patterned after the campaign of Hamilton Wright, FBN leaders were able to expand the negative feedback loop to include a new drug. All of the previous strategies of the moral entrepreneur were present: the sensationalist stories in the mass media, ideological contentions that marijuana led to the use of harder drugs and ultimately crimes of passion, and the rise of public sentiment against those who used the drug. Finally, there was the inevitable passage of federal legislation that enabled the FBN to control its use.

In order to set the stage for this legislation, a number of examples of typical marijuana-induced crimes were released to the mass media by the FBN. Some of the examples included the following:

In 1935, a 30-year old male assaulted a 10-year old girl, admitted being under the influence of marijuana, found to be crazy by the court and hanged.

In 1936, in San Antonio, Texas, two women were arrested for possession of marijuana and violently attacked the officer, C. Cullen. They were jailed.

In 1921, a male, 30 years old, beat to death with a rock a boy 14 years old while herding cattle in a pasture. He accused the boy of polluting his water supply and crushed his head and gouged out one eye before he fled the scene. He was arrested hours later at his home. He screamed and tore jail furniture and was found to be under the influence of marijuana. He was tried and hanged.

In 1933, in Tampa, Florida, a boy murdered his father, mother, and sister with an axe while under the influence of marijuana. He did not know of his actions until the next morning when he was arrested.[13]

Although there was little or no medical evidence to prove a causal relationship between the use of marijuana and specific acts of violence, there seems to have been little doubt in the minds of the legislators that marijuana should be controlled.[14] The public and governmental sentiments were further engaged through the distribution of a number of movies, including *Killer Weed* and *Assassin of Youth,* which depicted young and naive high school students being enticed into using the drug by unprincipled criminals. In the end the youths find only personal deterioration, crime, and insanity as the outcome of their actions.

By the time the Treasury Department went to the Congress with the marijuana tax bill, there was little doubt that the bill would be passed:

> Rather, the primary function of the hearing was to titillate the legislators with horror stories. They were assured that the act had the blessings of the newspapers. . . . The various crimes that the Bureau linked directly to marijuana were related, including the tale of the youngster who murdered his entire family while under the influence of marijuana. A district attorney told that the drug was an aphrodisiac, but prolonged use led to impotence. A pharmacologist . . . related that marijuana leads to mental and physical deterioration.
>
> The dissenting witnesses before the committee were limited. The birdseed industry feared that the new law would prohibit their use of hempseed. The committee quickly amended the bill to allow the industry to continue production.[15]

The tax act quickly passed the House and was sent on to the Senate, where it was passed within a short time.

The Marijuana Tax Act passed easily through the Congress primarily because of the FBN's previous legislative work at the state level. Like Wright before him, Anslinger devoted a considerable amount of time working between levels. Where Wright focused his campaign at the national level, giving him support at international conferences, Anslinger worked diligently at the state level to gain support for national legislation. The FBN actively cooperated with the National Conference of Commissioners on Uniform State Laws in developing uniform state regulations on narcotics and marijuana. From 1932 until 1937, the FBN made numerous reports to the conference indicating the need for stronger state legislation and implying that federal pressure might be brought to bear if the state did not act. In 1937, the FBN commented in its report, "The Federal Bureau of Narcotics can carry on no war of its own against this traffic.... The drug has come into wide and increasing abuse in many states, and the Bureau of Narcotics has therefore endeavored to impress upon the states the urgent need for vigorous enforcement of local cannabis laws."[16] By the time that the Marijuana Tax Act was passed (1937), most of the states had strict legislation prohibiting the production, use, sale, possession, and transportation of marijuana. Most also had outlawed the drug under the Bureau of Narcotics Uniform Narcotic Drug Act guidelines, which classified marijuana as an opiate. Although there is little clinical evidence to support this classification, the labelling of marijuana as a narcotic and the generation of enforcement policies that paralleled that of narcotics provided the public with the conception that something was being done to eradicate this problem.

In spite of the considerable appeal of the labelling approach, which sees the passage of this act as primarily the work of one man and his organization, recent conflict theorists have questioned whether one person really can amass that much power. As Collins notes, "No one man can unilaterally decide how large numbers of people will interact, and any pattern is the result of a struggle among many parties."[17] More recent research has indicated that this, in fact, was the case with the Marijuana Tax Act. Anslinger was certainly important at the organizational level, but his organization was riding a crest of negative public feeling against a certain group thought to use marijuana: the Mexicans.

A close scrutiny of the FBN publicity campaign against marijuana reveals that most of the bureau's public statements were made after the tax act was passed, between 1937 and 1939.[18] There is no doubt that Anslinger and his organization did their utmost to convince the public that this law was needed, but it seems that they had already gained the necessary political support for its passage and the campaign was designed more to quiet any remaining public doubts on the issue. The turn of events was not the moral entrepreneurs generating a mass media campaign that got the necessary public support for his legislation. Rather, the bureau had worked for many years with local, state, and national legislators, who were much more concerned with larger social issues, specifically the depression and aggravated racial tensions. The marijuana issue was a small side issue that fit into the larger pattern of racial domination.

Like the Chinese and blacks, who became the focus of antidrug legislation at the turn of this century, the Mexicans were visible, socially isolated, and perceived as a direct threat to significant groups within the larger society. Mexicans were visible not only because of their cultural differences and increased numbers but also because of the migratory nature of their work. Large numbers would drift into the rural small towns and work the fields during harvesttime and then migrate back to the large *barrios* in the cities during the off season. The nature of their work never let them become integrated into the larger communities but rather insured that they would remain culturally and politically isolated.

Of more significance to the fate of the Mexicans than either visibility or isolation was their location in the larger economic tensions of the Great Depression. Mexican labor was most useful to the large agribusiness of the Southwest that needed large groups of laborers during harvests but did not want to pay for their housing or social services during the off-seasons. If the large rural interests found the Mexicans necessary to their production processes, small farmers and urban interests found them a direct threat. After the start of the depression, small farmers in the West were being forced out of business by the larger and more efficient agribusinesses that employed Mexican labor.

Corporate agriculture was using the imported labor force not just to depress rural wage levels and lower unit costs in the short run but to finish off those traditional American ideals, the owner-operated family farm and the community of small but independent landowners, ideals that were already in a precarious economic position before the Depression.[19]

These groups, unable to ascertain the larger economic trends involved, vented their hostility on the Mexicans, who were making corporate profits possible.

Small farmers found an ally in the urban centers in the city officials who had to pay for public services for migrant workers during the off-season and in the urban laborers who competed with Mexicans for urban employment. "With the intensification of unemployment and the business losses of the thirties...[small farmers and urban interests made] a concrete, concerted effort at self-protection...[by] getting rid of the Mexicans."[20] These class tensions gave power to anti-Mexican feelings and stereotypes that portrayed Mexicans as essentially lazy, irresponsible, and prone toward using drugs and violent crime.

As long as the Mexicans were willing to work for the wages dictated by the growers and to live in economically squalid conditions, they did not threaten the growers' interests, and there was no significant criminal problem with Mexicans in these rural areas. According to a 1927 survey of Imperial County, the major agricultural section of southern California, "The record of law observances among Mexicans...is distinctly favorable to them."[21] A similar acknowledgment was made in rural areas of Texas and Colorado, where there was no mention of drug-induced crimes and no mention of marijuana at all.

In the cities, however, drug laws were a significant aspect of "the methods adopted for reducing the Mexican labor surplus in the city where surplus, and not scarcity as in the rural areas, was the fundamental economic threat."[22] The Mexicans tended to congregate in *barrios* in the major urban areas, making them targets for police persecution and harassment. Through intimidation and sporadic raids on these "high crime areas" inhabited by Mexicans, officials hoped to reduce the increasing influx of Mexicans into the cities. Although marijuana laws were a small part of this campaign, they did feed into the stereotype of the vicious drug-smoking menace of the inner city—the Mexican.

SOCIAL CONFLICT, BUREAUCRATIC CONTROL, AND THE RITUAL RESPONSE TO DRUG CRISIS

With the FBN's successful establishment of hegemony over the enforcement of drug laws, a peculiar organizational conflict inherent in all law enforcement agencies came to the fore. The ostensible reason for the organization's existence is to control and, implicitly, eliminate crime—in this case drug use. However, should the agency prove successful and eliminate crime, it also eliminates its legitimate basis for existence. Although the possibility of eliminating drug use is highly improbable, law enforcement agencies face a permanent and, ultimately, more insidious problem of institutional attrition. Resources are limited and must be spread among many federal agencies. To gain resources, an organization must appear to be highly effective, but it must not eliminate the food on which it feeds—in this case, lower-class drug users. The solution to the problem is periodic ritual "drug crises" in which the agency is seen to respond to an imminent threat. Once the threat has been removed, the bureau can request additional funds, go about its business, and wait for the next cycle. This is essentially the history of the FBN.

Faced with a long war of attrition that was never to be won, the structural interplay between drug users and the FBN was to remain somewhat consistent for almost four decades (1930 until 1968). During this period, the federal agency was content with a relatively mild system of cycles in which there would be a publicized increase in drug use followed by an effective law enforcement campaign and a degree of tranquility. The cycles ebbed approximately every fifteen years (1914, 1937, and 1949), and the federal bureaucracy would ride them out, expanding its influence, passing more stringent laws, and increasing its budget whenever possible.

During the thirty-year tenure of the FBN as the major drug enforcement agency, the bureau had been relatively successful in relegating drug use to certain specific subcultures. If the rise of narcotic legislation had found its impetus in the social conflict surrounding minority subcultures, the bureaucratic enforcement of these laws was no less narrowly confined. In the case of the opiates, the Harrison Act and subsequent state and local legislation was successful in confining its use to predominantly urban-based poor. After World War I, blacks had migrated from the rural South into the larger industrial cities of the Northeast and West looking for work. As the poor, unskilled blacks were relegated to both the least stable economic positions as well as forced into the most deteriorating sectors of the city, they conflicted with members of the white working classes who had originally occupied these economic and urban positions. Especially in the ethnic-dominated cities of New York and Chicago, tensions between the blacks and the foreign-born white workers increased, although some of the tension was dissipated as whites were able to move up economically and out geographically from the inner city. As the inner-city ghettos changed from Italian, Polish, and Jewish to black, this conflict motivated key political figures to search for an underlying cause for inner-city tensions, crime, and disorder. Characteristically, they looked to a drug conspiracy—a conspiracy supported by an emotional display coordinated by the FBN and a few key political figures, Senators Estes Kefauver and Congressman Hale Boggs.

As Collins pointed out, these displays are presented within the ecological context that dominates a particular period of history. In this case, America's newly won international position, derived from World War II, placed it at the forefront of the boundaries between the communist countries and the free world. It was a period of conspiracy theories run wild. Senator Joe McCarthy alleged he was finding communists in government, the movie industry, and even the army; Kefauver was finding an international conspiracy of Italians (Mafia) taking over the cities; and the FBN found both communists and the Mafia behind the rise in heroin addiction.

With China becoming communist in 1949, it was not difficult to tie the Chinese in the United States, the brunt of the early anti-opium crusade, with the international communist drug conspiracy. Anslinger spoke of the People's Republic of China as the definite point of origin for heroin and reported the arrest in Japan of "two or three Communist leaders for involvement in the traffic."[23] This statement before the influential Boggs Committee (the House Ways and Means Committee, Subcommittee on Drug Abuse, 1955, with responsibility for reforming drug laws) was reiterated before the United Nations three years later with the charges that the Chinese communist government was "distributing drugs abroad and . . . selling heroin and opium in large quantities to the free countries of the world." This trade, he claimed, generated the revenue that would be used "for political purposes and to finance agencies who have been found actively engaged" in the United States.[24]

Although research on the drugs that came to the United States from Asia indicates that it was not the communists but the Chinese

Nationalists, Thais, and Burmese who were behind the production and distribution this did not deter the government. With equal aplomb the Kefauver Committee, which was investigating organized crime, found a "tremendous flow" of marijuana and heroin into this country from Mexico under the direction of "some of the most astute, wiley, and desperate criminals who operate interstatewise."[25] With testimony from inner-city gang members, local and state officials, as well as the FBN, this committee concluded that organized crime was behind the apparent rise in drug use. Whether the source was an international political conspiracy (communism) or an international criminal conspiracy (Mafia), the solution was the same: strengthening the negative feedback loop with stiffer penalties.

Convinced that the answer to the drug problem was heavier penalties, the Congress authorized a minimum mandatory sentence of five years, with no chance of probation, suspended sentence, or parole and an optional fine of up to $20,000 for individuals convicted of selling narcotics, including marijuana. For persons convicted of possession of marijuana, the first offender faced a possible prison sentence of two to ten years with an optional fine of $20,000. The states followed suit, "Across the country state legislatures, most of them with small numbers of offenders to deal with, had followed the federal lead with 'little Boggs Acts.'"[26] Not only were penalties increased, but pressure was put on the courts to impose the full weight of these measures on the offenders.

The FBN's successful coordination of legislation with key members of the Congress was more a fine tuning of the social control process than a major expansion of the scope of the bureau's power over the drug issue. Whereas the Harrison Act and the Marijuana Tax Act were major legislative shifts toward the expansion of the bureau's discretionary power, this event had a more ritualistic air about it. However, it did act to solidify the FBN's status within the larger community of social control agencies. The display of conspiratorial agents at the center of the drug problem significantly supported a national ethos that buttressed political careers in the early 1950s. Kefauver became the Democratic vice-presidential candidate in 1952 while Boggs remained a powerful figure on Capitol Hill. Further, support from these influential congressional committees increased the FBN's public visibility and assured it a funding foundation for the next decade. Finally, the coordination of information between the state and federal drug enforcement agencies created avenues through which federal support for expanded narcotics enforcement at the local levels would be developed. By the mid-1950s, the FBN's stereotype of the dope fiend, its position as the source of accurate information, and its integration within the larger law enforcement community had been firmly established.

MINORITIES, MUSIC, AND INFORMATIONAL MAYHEM: THE BLURRING OF THE BUREAUCRATIC DOCTRINE ON DRUGS

The history of drug enforcement thus far has reflected the steady advances of the FBN over minority subcultures through the use of a number of organizational strategies. Specifically, the bureau was initially created and later advanced its organizational interests through the control of conferences in which the problematic nature of drug use was structured into a stereotype, the presentation of this stereotype in emotional displays for public consumption, the control of legal ambiguities to increase organizational power, and the generation of reciprocal interdependence with important government committees for the maintenance and advancement of organizational power. The key factor that runs through much of the FBN's organizational strategy has been the attempt to control information in a manner that would solidify the negative feedback loop. Throughout the history of the bureau, this strategy has effectively coincided with public and congressional fears of minority groups that have evolved out of larger social and economic tensions. The bureau effectively rode the sentiments of the day and built more salience into the social control system that was ostensibly aimed at curtailing drug use but was ultimately effective in oppressing minorities.

The bureau's hegemony was due largely to the increased bifurcation between the deviant groups and the larger middle-class society. Because the split between minorities and whites was well developed throughout the first six decades of this century, there was little possibility of the rise of an alternative definition and a subsequent positive feedback loop. During the decades between the initial establishment of drug enforcement agencies under the Harrison Act and the FBN reorganization in 1967, drug users were socially isolated, culturally stigmatized, and politically impotent. It was only with the rise of massive cultural shifts between the dominant middle class and minorities that the bureau's stereotype came under serious attack.

The stereotype of the dope fiend describes an individual who is lethargic, undisciplined, and prone to violence. Although this stereotype met little resistance among members of the middle class, there were groups who used drugs and enjoyed a degree of public appreciation. During the 1930s, 1940s, and 1950s, some prominent members of the entertainment business, especially musicians, used drugs to heighten their creative powers. Although some used heroin, marijuana was a much more common supplement to the alcohol that flowed during all-night jam sessions in the bars of major American cities. As Mexican-Americans moved into the cities in the 1930s, it was not long before inner-city blacks found marijuana compatible with their life-style, especially the life-style of the jazz musician.

In this case, marijuana was used to increase one's ability to decipher music, spontaneously create new forms of music in jam sessions, and play an instrument in a "hotter" manner. The jazz musician saw himself as self-consciously outside the mainstream of society, "as an artist who possesses a mysterious artistic gift setting him apart from all other people. Possessing this gift, he should be free from control by outsiders who lack it. . . . Under no circumstances should any outsider be allowed to tell him what to play or how to play it."[27] This attitude, coupled with the use of marijuana, put the musical subculture in direct opposition to legal authorities entrusted with the control of the drug. The *Minneapolis Tribune* reflected this in an article stating that federal narcotics agents were aware that "present day swing music, the Big Apple Dance, and orchestra jam sessions are responsible for increasing the use of marijuana, both by dance band musicians and by the boys and girls who patronize them."[28]

Although there was considerable tension between these two groups and numerous charges and countercharges of drug use by musicians were made, most persons arrested for drug use were relatively minor musicians. The major bands—those of Count Basie, Louis Armstrong, the Dorsey Brothers, Dizzy Gillespie, and Lionel Hampton— did not run into direct confrontation from officials, but all had been investigated by the FBN. After World War II, Harry Anslinger made a special effort to infiltrate the musician subculture and to prosecute anyone on whom he could get substantial information. The ethic of the subculture, however, made it next to impossible to get informants and generate a substantial case. Since he could not generate a case that would be viable in court, he then attempted to get the State Department to revoke the passport of musicians thought to be using the drug and influencing Europeans in its use. The State Department rejected this idea as too vague, and Anslinger was unable to close a case on any major musician. Although the FBN had found legislative bodies amenable to coordinated attacks on the drug issue, law enforcement agents—in this case the State Department—were less than enthusiastic. As Collins suggests, "The more initiative required in a task, and the less predictable or visible the outcomes, the more its successful accomplishment depends on strong normative controls."[29] Obviously, the expansion of the area of drug control by the moral entrepreneur is an excellent example of the need for individual initiative in an area not completely predictable. Further, "the more exclusive the emphasis on normative control, the more likely there are to be intense factional conflicts at policy-making levels."[30] Anslinger and the State Department were engaged in a factional conflict on the proper normative approach to law enforcement that would become the watchword for much of the bureau's enforcement efforts. There is often intense organizational conflict among law enforcement agencies on the proper procedures to curtail the drug problem. In this case, the possible use of marijuana by musicians was not enough of an issue in the eyes of the State Department to warrant the procedures the FBN desired.

Creative artists also used cocaine but not as consistently as marijuana. Whereas marijuana was often the domain of black, and often poor, musicians, cocaine was the drug of the upper classes and especially the fast-paced Hollywood set. This was true in the 1920s, during prohibition, when many people had found cocaine a pleasant addition to their life-styles. However, the new legal constraints created a black market that drove prices up. People of means found it more feasible to use cocaine because they could afford to visit a doctor or get a prescription that provided legal access to the drug. The few studies of cocaine addiction during this period indicate that many users were from the professional classes.

Not only middle-class professionals but a number of well-known actors and members of the upper classes are known to have used the drug privately or introjected references to the drug into their movies during this period. Tallulah Bankhead, Cole Porter, Fatty Arbuckle, and Charlie Chaplin were thought to have used cocaine. This is seen in the Charlie Chaplin movie *Modern Times*, where Chaplin is in mortal opposition to the menace of industrial life, especially the factory. He takes a few snorts from a "mysterious white powder" and proceeds to destroy the aggravating technological monster. Although *Modern Times* was first shown in 1936, "the very fact that Chaplin felt able to use such a reference in the mid-thirties ... indicates that either it was so widely known to the masses a few years earlier that no one had forgotten it, or that Chaplin believed its prevalence in Hollywood reflected a nationwide pattern."[31]

The popularity of cocaine soon diminished, not to arise again until the early 1970s. With the depression of the 1930s and the increased pressure on drugs by the federal government after the repeal of prohibition in 1933, cocaine tended to recede from the popular consciousness. By 1931 every state had severe criminal penalties for all but medical use of the drug. Also the FBN increased its surveillance of the importation of coca leaves, making it difficult to divert the drug from these legitimate sources into the black market. Probably the most significant cause of the decline in cocaine use was the introduction of amphetamines in 1932. These stimulants proved to be cheaper, longer lasting, and more available to the public. The increased price and difficulty in buying cocaine made it much less popular as a recreational drug.

If drug use was confined primarily to minorities and musicians in the decades preceding the late 1960s, this trend met with an intense and rapid transition between 1965 and 1970. Just as the antidrug legislation was a reflection of much larger social transformations, so the transformation of these laws and the agencies developed for their enforcement can be traced to deeper social issues. It was the stable bifurcation of minorities from the dominant middle-class society that enabled the drug stereotype to persist unchallenged. However, the cultural, social, and political upheaval of the late 1960s created the inroads for information flow between the two groups.

Just as the moral entrepreneur had manipulated the mass media to coordinate the construction of the dope fiend stereotype, the mass media became the channel through which new white and minority perspectives were structured. The stereotype of the lazy, undisciplined black or Chicano was confronted with media images of black power and *Viva la raza*. What had been dirty, lazy, and cowardly Chinese at the turn of the century and an international communist conspiracy in the early 1950s was now a major world power and, for some, a model of the new social order. Racial turmoil within the United States, the war in Vietnam, and a booming economy at home created the conditions for the reversal of the drug fiend stereotype. If the economic downturn and split labor force created the rise of antidrug legislation, the increased affluence and political attempts at integrating the labor force reversed it. The late 1960s and early 1970s was a period of economic optimism, a mood felt the strongest in the idealism and rejection of materialism that typified many of the youth of that period. Born in the 1940s, they missed the pressure of the depression and viewed middle-class materialism, caution, and desire for upward social mobility as suspect. This cultural shift was aggravated by the proportionately large number of individuals in this group. The baby boom of the post-World War II period created a major influx of students into American colleges. The relative independence, tendency toward liberal ideals, and large numbers of these individuals made them a force to reckon with—a reckoning that was felt by drug enforcement agencies.

The social factors were there: economic prosperity, a tendency toward liberal experimentation, increased empathy for previously stigmatized groups, and a disillusionment with past values. In these respects, there were fewer normative pressures on these individuals than was the case on most of their parents or older siblings. The final element was a new form of information control, a new stage on which an emotional display could be performed to establish a new definition and concomitant information loop. The new moral entrepreneur was a young, Irish, Harvard University psychologist and, like his forerunners, he presented a charismatic image on which others could be moved to adopt a new view of the reality of drugs.

If Wright and Anslinger used their institutional groundings to legitimate their views, Doctors Timothy Leary and Richard Alpert gained their initial public focus from Harvard University. In conducting a number of experiments on the effects of marijuana, they "used far more subjects than any other marijuana research . . . and had their subjects take [the drug] under natural conditions of environment . . .

something which had never been done before."[32] This research met with initial encouragement from the scientific community. Leary and Alpert were also doing research on a little-known but extremely powerful drug, LSD.

There had been little objective research on drugs until 1965, but there have been several more philosophical positions expounded by literary figures of the time. Just as the nineteenth-century men of letters presented a problematic view of opium and initiated the negative feedback loop, the Harvard psychologist, coupled with a number of eminent philosophers, set the stage for a positive definition of LSD. Specifically, Aldous Huxley, probably one of the most well-known American writers, had a deep interest in Eastern religion. His intellectual interest in this area was combined with deep personal experiences with mescaline, a drug similar to LSD. In a book that was widely read in the late 1960s, *Doors to Perception*, Huxley presents a strong case for the religious potential of this chemical. He wrote:

Mescaline raises all colours to a higher power and makes the percipient aware of innumerable fine shades of difference, to which, at ordinary times, he is completely blind.... Like mescaline takers, many mystics perceive supernaturally brilliant colours, not only with the inward eye, but even in the objective world around them. Similar reports are made by psychics and sensitives.[33]

In a manner reminiscent of Freud's descriptions of cocaine, he expounded the virtues of mescaline over the more traditional drugs:

To most people, mescaline is almost completely innocuous. Unlike alcohol, it does not drive the taker into a...brawl. A man under the influence of mescaline [has] experiences of the most enlightening kind.... Although obviously superior to cocaine, opium, alcohol and tobacco...its effects last for an inconveniently long time.... If the psychologist and the sociologist will define the ideal [of transcendence through chemistry], the neurologist and pharmacologist can be relied upon to discover the means whereby that ideal can be realized.[34]

When Huxley wrote these words in 1954, he had no idea that he was forecasting the events that were to take place some twenty years later.

The next major proponent of the drug culture was Alan Watts, an ex-Episcopalian priest who had become widely regarded as one of the foremost scholars on Eastern religion. Watts lived on a houseboat across San Francisco Bay in Sausalito and gained a wide following among both scholars and young people interested in altered states of consciousness. Watts wrote over thirty books on Eastern thought, but the most significant one to influence the drug culture was *The Joyous Cosmology*. In this work he, like Huxley, described his experiences with psychoactive drugs in extraordinary terms:

> For quite suddenly I feel my understanding dawning into a colossal clarity, as if everything were opening up down to the roots of my being and of time and space themselves. The sense of the world becomes totally obvious. I am struck with amazement that I or anyone could have thought life a problem or mystery. I call everyone to gather around.... Listen, I have something to tell.[35]

And tell he did. Some of the first to listen were Leary and Alpert. They wrote the introduction to *The Joyous Cosmology* and gave these views, at least to the nonacademic layman, an initial aura of respectability. Leary and Alpert tried to integrate their experimental findings on LSD with

> conventional models of western psychology ... psychoanalytic, behavioristic ... and found these concepts quite inadequate to map the richness and breadth of expanding consciousness.... We have had to return again and again to the nondualistic conceptions of eastern philosophy, a theory of mind made more explicit and familiar in our western world by Bergson, Aldous Huxley, and Alan Watts.[36]

If opium and cocaine were initially defined in terms of the predominant values of the late nineteenth century (reduction of pain, creation of an energized normal state), the psychedelic drugs (mescaline, psilocybin, and LSD) were initially legitimated with references to Eastern Religion. Just as the men of letters during the nineteenth century told of unbound joy, strength, and visions from opium and cocaine, so the new chemical substances on the mid-twentieth century road to nirvana had equally fantastic billing. The high priests of the new culture had been named, the sacraments had been identified, and the norms had been outlined; all that was needed were the parishioners.

This general ideological setting, coupled with the social and economic trends toward affluence and liberalism, made it possible for small pockets of a new drug culture to form. It was not surprising that the most intense development of this culture came on the West Coast, especially in San Francisco, where Far Eastern culture is strongest and cultural diversity is most tolerated.[37] An area known as the Haight-Ashbury district in the western part of San Francisco and Telegraph Avenue in Berkeley became the colonies for this rising social movement. By 1967, these urban areas were the undisputed centers for the "hippie" movement. However, in every major city young people would frequent the shops that sold drug paraphernalia, colorful posters, and drug literature. These areas were also the location for illicit street drug traffic and sometimes rock concerts.

Of less intensity but still of significant influence was the Greenwich Village area of New York City where the "beats" of the 1950s took their stand. As the 1960s wore on, many of the young hip people of this area moved into the poorer sections of the East Village and the Lower East Side. As the young whites spread into these sections of the city, they mingled more with minorities, groups that earlier had received much vilification for taking drugs. If San Francisco and New York were the initial points of the hippie movement, Los Angeles was the mecca for those who desired commercial success with the new rock sound that was evolving out of the drug culture. Although minorities did not intermingle much with the Los Angeles-Sunset Boulevard scene, many who had spent time in the other two cities came there in hopes of commercial success. As they came, they brought the new message expounded by Leary concerning drug use: "tune in, turn on, and drop out." The message found fertilization in the debris of the inner cities where minorities had tuned out, turned off, and had no choice but to stay out for years. Now, respectable middle-class, usually well-educated youth freely invaded the urban ghettos to find peace, love, and cosmic joy through the new world of chemistry. If the medical association had been imbued with the Pollyanna principle in terms of cocaine and heroin, the youth culture took it to its logical extreme—a way of life premised on drug use.

The avenues on which the street scene flourished in the late 1960s provided a number of social functions for the rise and dissemination of a new feedback loop on drug use. "Most important, the Avenue functions to keep the colony [of drug users] together. Information is passed along about absent friends or partners, new people in town, events in San Francisco, and on college campuses, and especially the activities of the police."[38] This closely knit, oral social structure quickly developed an in-group identity that insulated it from the outside world of nondrug users. It also expanded the positive definition of drug use into new groups of outsiders. These urban colonies acted as the generators and initial disseminators of a feedback loop that would successfully undermine much of the FBN's carefully structured view on drug use.

Although "it appear[ed] that drug use will not only encourage a person to participate in some new scene, but it will ... [make a] deeply involved ... drug user ... less likely to associate with 'straight' people."[39] The street scenes and their surrounding colonies acted as a location in which individuals could experiment with psychoactive drugs, interaction among members could generate a new and intense cultural system, and, most importantly, the culture could be disseminated throughout the country.

In a strange twist, the mass media, once deeply influenced by the government bureau in the area of drug information, became a sounding board for those who favored drugs as a major part of their life-style; television and magazine coverage of the hippies became commonplace. The most effective tool for spreading the new gospel was records. Between 1966 and 1969, recording stars generated a number of records that told of the joys of drug use, initially LSD, marijuana and, by the early 1970s, cocaine. The radio played songs like "Lucy in the Sky with Diamonds" by the Beatles. Country Joe and the Fish imposed background voices saying "LSD" in their songs, and the Jefferson Airplane made explicit references to "magic mushrooms" (psilocybin) in their records. This emphasis on psychedelic drugs was relatively short-lived (1966–1970), but it was the wedge that eventually opened the gates for the popularization of other drugs.

This psychedelic wedge was ideological in nature and had very little to do with the effects of the drug on its users. Of all of the drugs to become popular in the country, LSD was probably the least predictable and the most potent. As one researcher put it:

Most subjects find the experience valuable, some find it frightening, and many say it is uniquely lovely.... For myself, my experiences with these substances have been the most strange, awesome, and among the most beautiful things in a varied and fortunate life. These are not escapes from, but enlargements, burgeonings of reality.[40]

The fact that "most subjects found the experience valuable" is indicated by the massive increase in drug use within the middle classes. However, the existential possibility of "the bad trip" always lurked.

It was not the drug experience that gave the movement its influence but the whole cultural ethos and its ability to become surreptitiously infused into the nondrug-using culture through the mass media. Whether through formal advocacy, as in the case of Huxley, Watts, or Leary and Alpert, or in a less forthright manner by the lyrics of rock music, the new definition of drug use began to circulate before the federal government was aware of it. The psychedelic revolution had begun and the FBN found itself on the ideological defensive for the first time in almost forty years. The new commissioner of the FBN, who had replaced Anslinger in 1960, stated to the congressional subcommittee on drugs:

Within the past few years we have witnessed a dramatic increase in drug abuse throughout the United States, primarily among young people. . . . The most dramatic increase seems to have occurred in the abuse of so-called hallucinogenic drugs, primarily LSD and marijuana.[41]

There is no doubt about the authenticity of the rise of drug use, but a major problem faced the bureau: how to interpret this new phenomenon. Evidence indicates that this new form of drug use did not fit the FBN stereotype of the individual progressively moving from alcohol, to marijuana, to heroin. Rather, research on the street scenes indicates little interest in heroin.[42] A further problem came in the interpretation of marijuana, which had been classified along with opium and heroin but was now labelled as "hallucinogenic" or, on the street, a psychedelic drug. The bureau also recognized the influence of the hippie culture in this rise of drug use but was not easily able to integrate this new cultural context into their old stereotype.[43]

In an almost ritualistic manner, the government took a punitive stance on this issue and moved toward enacting strict legal penalties against the new threat (LSD). A law was passed that made the "illegal sale, distribution, manufacture, or possession [of LSD]...a felony punishable by up to five years imprisonment."[44] In a style established by the bureau during the 1930s and revived in the early 1950s, the FBN commissioner stated that "the link between marijuana and heroin has been firmly established, and many authorities also agree that there is a definite association between marijuana and LSD abuse."[45] This statement reflects the notion of a linear continuum of drug use, implicitly beyond the willful control of the user, which leads many from simple experimentation to addiction and degradation. "A penalty against unauthorized possession is necessary," the commissioner believed, "since it deters use of drugs by countless persons who might otherwise be tempted to experiment, often with disastrous consequences."[46] Although the validity of this view was never accurately determined, there is considerable evidence that this traditional drug ideology was not being accepted by the drug subculture or by an increasing portion of nonusers.[47] The FBN's emotional display was not penetrating the new stage of the hippie minority, their music, and the resulting informational mayhem.

Although LSD and marijuana acted as a wedge to break up the government's monopoly on information control, the extreme diversity of reactions to LSD reduced its positive image within the drug subculture. However, by the early 1970s, the underground had successfully revived a drug that was either too expensive or had been effectively controlled by the FBN: cocaine. In a manner reminiscent of the late 1960s, rock stars began inserting mention of the drug into their lyrics. The Rolling Stones, the Grateful Dead, the Jefferson Airplane, and others all made explicit references to "coke," as did folk and country western artists. Johnny Cash, one of the most popular country-western singers, sang of his "Cocaine Blues" in 1969 ("Lay off the whiskey and let that cocaine be"). Lesser known but no less subtle references to cocaine were made by Hoyt Axton ("Snow Blind Friend") and Laura Nyro ("Buy and Sell"). Movies, such as the extremely popular *Easy Rider* and *Superfly* glamorized the free and easy coke dealer. Although these aspects of the pop culture have come and gone, they did sensitize the drug subculture to cocaine as a new means for personal pleasure.

The rapid rise of cocaine in the early 1970s can be traced to the force of the newly formed positive definition of drug use. Further, the feedback loop between users and nonusers was expansive enough to support the introduction of many drugs into the middle classes. What had been a drug culture based on LSD and marijuana in the late 1960s had been diffused, both in the type of person using drugs and the kind of drugs used. By the early 1970s, the drug street scene had all but disappeared. The psychedelic culture had quickly ebbed and flowed, in a much more diluted form, into the suburbs. As Douglas found in his 1973 study,

> The rapid decline of the street scene does not mean that there has been any decrease in the number of drug users or in the amount of drugs taken. ... Clearly LSD is no longer the fad drug it was in the middle and later 1960's at the height of the street scene. The new fads have been cocaine, hashish, and, more recently, methaqualones [Sopors and Quaaludes, for example]. But these fads are laid over the earlier ones, rather than replacing them."[48]

Drug use was a common, and mostly accepted, aspect of middle American culture.

Although drug use is not legally condoned, only the most visible violations are sanctioned. The FBN's negative definition of heroin has remained strong, primarily because of the drug's powerful addictive capacity. However, marijuana, cocaine, methaqualones, and, to a significantly diminished extent, the hallucinogens enjoy a relatively positive or neutral social definition. Rather than a distinct social demarcation between drug user and nonuser, they exist amicably together in most all social contexts. On the whole, the same factors that created the negative feedback loop at the turn of the century were responsible for its demise in the late 1960s. Specifically, the decline of minority isolation and the affluence of the period allowed for more cultural flexibility between these groups. The affluence gave middle-class youth the opportunity to experiment with new life-styles, one of which was to generate a minority status based on drugs. Hippie youth was a category between the "dope fiend" and the respectable middle-class adolescent. They fit all of the characteristics of the dope fiend but never lost their middle-class roots. Those who had dropped out in the late 1960s, unlike their minority forebears, could rejoin the main-stream at their discretion. When they did this, they brought their life-style with them.

REACTION AND REORGANIZATION: THE BUREAUCRATIC
RESPONSE TO THE NEW DEFINITION OF DRUG USE

The late 1960s had generated a new positive and pervasive feedback loop between drug users and nonusers that significantly undermined the views presented by the FBN. This period not only created an external pressure on the bureau, but a number of internal tensions were also being felt. The historical context in which drug legislation was developed administratively divided the drug enforcement process between two separate federal agencies. Narcotics law enforcement had developed under the Treasury Department in the form of the FBN, with the Customs Bureau and Coast Guard playing subsidiary roles. However, synthetic drugs that had been developed in the 1930s were controlled within the Department of Health, Education and Welfare (HEW). If the American Medical Association had lost its fight with the FBN over opium, cocaine, and marijuana, it was strong enough by the 1930s to have these drugs controlled by a less stringent administrative system. The amphetamines, barbiturates, and other synthetic drugs were controlled by physicians under the administrative guidelines of HEW, and little was made of their potential for abuse within the mass media. However, with the rise of the drug culture in the late 1960s, the political pressure for increased law enforcement was pervasive enough to require a reorganization of this dual structure.

This political reaction and movement for administrative reform was also manifest within the FBN itself. The feelings of many who had either observed or worked within the bureau were echoed by John Ingersoll, the head of the reorganized version of the FBN. Ingersoll and other reformers felt that

corruption had reached high levels [within the FBN].... Key informants were killed. Other law enforcement organizations did not trust the FBN.... Informants had too much freedom and too much control over who was going to be arrested. ... There was no particular security over the files that revealed the identity of informants.[49]

There are two interrelated sources of this organizational malaise: the quality of the agents within the organization and the nature of the law enforcement task. Throughout the Bureau's history, it had been difficult to find individuals who would be eager to engage in the often dangerous work of uncovering narcotics traffic. But the former commissioner "took what he could find, happy if one out of every fifth agent hired proved to be honest, fairly efficient, and loyal."[50] The nature of the work involved long hours, working within one of the most dangerous environments in law enforcement, and received little in the way of public recognition. Compared to the counterparts in the FBI, narcotics agents and their work were less than the pinnacle of the law enforcement hierarchy.

With the rise of drug use, the bifurcated drug enforcement structure, and increased criticism from within, the time was ripe for reorganization. It came in two waves. The first involved Reorganization Plan I (1967) in which the FBN and HEW drug control agency were merged into the Bureau of Narcotics and Dangerous Drugs (BNDD). It was clear to the initial organizers of this new bureau that effective control of drugs would require the centralization of decision making, a broadening of administrative scope to include all major drugs, and, most importantly, the integration of information flow to this centralized agency. Along with the rise of drug use came new definitions of drug use, amorphous webs of drug distribution on the streets, and the rise of new international smuggling organizations. The control of information in each of these areas was central to combating this new problem.

The second wave of reaction and reorganization came six years later, in 1973, when President Nixon created the Drug Enforcement Agency (DEA) out of the BNDD. This second reorganization was a further attempt to centralize all government bureaus having any function related to drugs into one comprehensive agency. Under Reorganization Plan I, the FBN had been integrated with the HEW enforcement unit into one unified domestic control agency. However, drug interdiction at the international border was still the responsibility of Customs, Immigration and Naturalization, and the Coast Guard. After six years of increasing drug use in the United States, President Nixon declared war on the international drug traffic and called it America's number one problem.

As had been the case throughout the history of drug enforcement, power comes with information control. As Collins suggests, "The more efficient the technology of transportation and communication, the more central control can be maintained in a situation of large size and geographical dispersion."[51] Large size and geographical dispersion certainly describes the border area around the continental United States. It includes more than 15,000 miles of desert, mountains, and ocean. There are over 600 ports of entry through which federal officials attempt to funnel, inspect, and apprehend smugglers. There are vast areas between these ports through which smugglers use increasingly sophisticated cars, boats, and airplanes to bring drugs into the country. As one federal report summarized, "Quality intelligence concerning the activities of smugglers, in combination with mobile, air, water, or ground interception, is considered to be the best tool to improve interdiction results, short of total surveillance" of the border area.[52]

The history of drug enforcement bureaus has been one in which power has self-consciously expanded into areas of organizational ambiguity. The overlapping and often conflicting attempts to control international drug traffic by several federal agencies seems to reflect a considerable amount of such ambiguity.

The stage was set, and the DEA created its master plan. Specifically, it enlisted members of each of the organizations entrusted with some aspect of border interdiction who had spent at least 50 percent of their time in the area of drug control. The DEA was composed of members of Customs, the Immigration and Naturalization Service (INS), the Coast Guard, and to a lesser extent, the FBI and Federal Aeronautics Administration (FAA). The DEA also generated an overall strategy that emphasized an incremental approach. The DEA agents worked with local, state, and international drug control agencies and gathered information to be integrated into DEA computers. This information system would become the basis for focusing undercover work to set up a particular suspect. Once arrested, this suspect was pressured to assist DEA agents in setting up his supplier, who would then go through the same ordeal. Eventually, it was believed, the DEA would be able to work its way up into the highest echelons of the drug trafficking business.

Few other federal agencies felt particularly threatened by this new, well-publicized agency. Most had developed a record of effectiveness within their area of expertise and did not need the added burden of drug raids to upgrade their organizational image. The FAA, INS,

Coast Guard, and FBI were fully occupied controlling air traffic, illegal aliens, sea commerce, and criminals within the United States. However, with Customs, the smooth road toward the co-optation of organizational ambiguity met with some less than ambiguous resistance. Customs had enjoyed a considerable amount of discretionary power over international interdiction, especially between 1967 and 1973, when the intranational BNDD was the central drug control agency. As the DEA spread its organizational tentacles over this area previously controlled by Customs, considerable interorganizational conflict arose.

The conflict centered on differences between these agencies over organizational strategies and the role of information within each strategic system. As Customs Commissioner Agee stated to the U.S. Congressional Subcommittee on Drug Control:

At our borders it [drugs] crosses in its greatest purity and its greatest bulk because, once it hits the domestic side, falls into the domestic distribution pattern, it literally is scattered to the winds. And to try and work it back from the street level to the lowest distribution level to the middle distribution level and back to the border again is almost an impossible task.[53]

Whereas the DEA felt that working up from the bottom of the drug distribution system would generate positive results in the long run. Customs saw it as an "impossible task," believing that the most fruitful approach was to tap it at the point of greatest bulk and purity, a point in the distribution system dominated by Customs.

It was not that Customs was opposed to a centralized system of information gathering and coordination. Rather, Customs felt it to be more efficient to retain the existing Customs operation and have the DEA system work with rather than displace Customs. Interagency tensions focused most intensely on the DEA's construction of a new computer system for border interdiction at El Paso, Texas. The El Paso Information Center (EPIC) was designed to integrate all drug information available from all border agencies, but, in Customs's view, it simply displaced their already existing system.

The Customs system, Treasury Enforcement Communications System (TECS), had computer terminals at all of the border ports of entry, international airports, and sea ports. Headquartered in San

Diego, TECS boasted a total of 485,000 records, with 220,000, or 45 percent, being drug related. Further, the system had been integrated with both local and state law enforcement agencies, as well as with the FBI's National Crime Information Center.[54] In the six years (1967–1973) that Customs had hegemony over the structuring of information related to drug smuggling, it began to develop a well-integrated and comprehensive communication network. It was becoming integrated with national law enforcement agencies and had also made contact, if somewhat imperfectly, with foreign customs units. The Mexican and Canadian agencies were most relevant for drug interdiction, but the larger international information network was also important. The U.S. Customs service has been "a member of the Customs Cooperation Council, headquartered in Brussels...an eighty nation organization.... [Further, this is an effective network because] Customs people speak the same language, whether it be in New York or Rome or Brussels or whatever."[55] Customs had used the six years effectively by generating an integrated national, as well as the beginnings of an international, information network designed to facilitate drug interdiction at the borders. In short, Customs had already developed the efficient technology of communication and was not interested in giving up its central control over this area of drug enforcement.

The DEA, with its new presidentially ordained mission and a sizable budget, was effectively encroaching on a system already developed by Customs. Customs, on the defensive, turned to the ritualized stage of congressional hearings in an effort to present an emotional display. It was necessary to prove that their strategy and technical support system was more effective than that of the DEA. In a double-edged statement, Customs Commissioner Agee stated to the House Subcommittee on Drug Traffic that "since reorganization, we have been dependent on DEA to provide [Customs] with information and it simply has not been forthcoming because they don't have it to provide."[56] When queried as to whether the DEA was being uncooperative, he answered that the agency was cooperating with Customs, but he implied that the lack of forthcoming information indicated administrative incompetence, an incompetence not reflected in Customs's information-gathering structure. The commissioner went on to state that "a recent [1976] analysis of narcotics seizures [at the border] discloses that less than one percent of all narcotics seizures [made by Customs in that year] were based upon prior information from DEA."[57]

Unlike the different drug enforcement agencies (FBN, BNDD, and now DEA), Customs was not interested in displacing other agencies and was actually supportive of DEA's general strategy and its international information network. Drugs were only one form of contraband crossing the international border and, from Customs's view, they were willing to work with the DEA as long as the latter left border interdiction primarily to them. Customs had an international connection with its Mexican counterpart and was not disturbed that the DEA had developed ties with Mexican authorities who specialized in drug traffic control. Customs, nevertheless, did point out bureaucratic ineptness on several fronts. Specifically, the DEA seemed to have communication problems within its own agency. The DEA-Mexican information network, Interdepartmental Intelligence Group-Mexico (IDIG-M), was based in Washington but had little interaction with the DEA's border system, EPIC. The commissioner stated that "EPIC and IDIG-M remain two separate efforts to deal with the Mexican narcotics problem. But even though they are under the leadership of the DEA, neither communicate to combine their efforts."[58] Not only was the DEA expanding into an area that was already operating under Customs, but, from Customs's view, it was expanding at such a rate that it was not able to remain internally integrated. The DEA had neither effectively integrated itself with foreign enforcement agencies nor created the centralized information system within the United States for its own operational effectiveness.

But Customs was willing to "compromise":

Under a single agency inspection system, each screening location [port of entry, airport, and so forth] would have a terminal to access simultaneously the complete file of all relevant information.... Obviously, compared to current plans [to expand the DEA's EPIC system] a jointly used system [DEA in Washington and Customs controlling the border] offers significant reduction in resource outlays for computers, related telecommunication, and possibly inspector processing time.[59]

That is, DEA could continue its overall strategy of an integrated international telecommunication system that would be the basis for working up its drug arrest system. Customs could then concentrate on the border interdiction efforts, and each agency could exchange information. In this way Customs would retain discretionary hegemony on its information and arrest process.

During the 1970s, the newly formed DEA was having its share of problems too. It was faced with a nationally publicized drug problem, considerable intra-agency confusion, and a sizable amount of hostility from established enforcement agencies that feared encroachment. The best this new agency could do was present a positive image to the key congressional committees and work to integrate its system as quickly as possible. In terms of the accusations from Customs, the DEA commissioner stated to the congressional committee that "as far as I am concerned, any information they need is theirs for the asking and I have so instructed my people."[60] He further indicated that the information network with Mexico was improving: "The overall Mexican . . . enforcement situation, I would say, looks encouraging. I have just met with the Attorney General of Mexico and he indicates that the Mexican Government will continue to cooperate on drugs and continue this program."[61]

These optimistic views, however, were countered by the government's watchdog agency, the Government Accounting Office (GAO). In a study made during 1975, the GAO found that during the six-month period between November 1975 and May 1976, the DEA sent sixty-four memorandums to the Mexican intelligence units but received only three in return.[62] The DEA was coming under fire from a number of government agencies, and the tensions would not diminish. Customs rejuvenated its efforts to prove its organizational superiority over the DEA and regain its operational hegemony. To do this, it went on the offensive in 1976 in an effort to organize border information and interdiction efforts under its own organizational structure. The DEA's weak initial performance at the border created a problematic situation, which Customs set out to exploit.

If the history of narcotics enforcement has been one of organizational expansion through the domination of areas of ambiguity, Customs was no less inclined toward this strategy than were its DEA adversaries. Customs decided to take the offensive and demonstrate its organizational effectiveness by generating three operations in which Customs was the coordinating agency and in charge of the communication network. Ostensibly these operations would reestablish communication and operational links with other agencies, raise the status of Customs closer to its previous position, and possibly reduce the onslaught of bureaucratic power from the heavily funded DEA. However, this strategy proved less than completely effective.

The first operation, entitled Diamondback, took place along the Mexican-Texan border and included the DEA, the INS, the FAA, and the Coast Guard. Each of these agencies was to be an equal partner under the general coordinating efforts of the Customs. The operation lasted for over a month in the spring of 1976 and proved to be more of an embarrassment than a coup for Customs. Many of the criticisms that Customs had leveled at the DEA returned to haunt Customs when this program was evaluated by its participants. "Fundamental planning and coordination of the operation never got out of the idea stage.... Intelligence data to field units from headquarters or command level was nonexistent."[63] A memorandum to Customs from the Coast Guard stated that "this operation was rushed into execution with little or no planning at the field level and consequently was fraught with many flaws."[64] Ultimately, in terms of actual contraband being detected and confiscated, even Customs acknowledged that the operation was a failure. Only in ground operations, especially at the ports of entry where Customs had already generated a smooth operation, were any drugs found. Air and sea operations were a failure, no arrests and seizures were made.

The other two operations, Star Trek I and II, took place along the California-Arizona and Mexico borders and involved the same group of federal border agencies. Unlike operation Diamondback, in which Customs was both the major coordinating and information disseminating agency, Customs decided to make DEA responsible for disseminating data, realizing that a more modest organizational goal for the second operation would be in its best interest. And so it was. This time, DEA took the criticism for poor information management, while Customs could take the credit for an overall increase in drugs confiscated. Customs reported that "scant information was provided by DEA" during the fifty-two days of operation. In spite of this poor cooperation, Customs claimed that the operation had been a genuine success. Each of the Star Trek operations confiscated at least twice as much marijuana as operation Diamondback had and a considerable amount of cocaine and heroin, none of which was found at the first operation.[65] The DEA countered against the Customs image of organizational efficiency by stating that it "only received two telephone calls from Star Trek personnel during the operation."[66]

It is difficult to determine whether Customs administrators consciously attempted to embarrass the DEA by making it responsible for information dissemination and then informally cutting it out of the operation. On the other hand, interagency rivalry may have been so intense that agents at all levels of each organization tended to eschew communications with their counterparts in the other organization. Irrespective of the organizational source for the conflict, whether a decision at the top or diffuse tensions throughout each structure, the results were the same: interorganizational conflict, an ineffective pooling of resources, and a general lack of support from those who evaluated these operations.

Specifically, "over the past few years the Congress, the executive branch, and the GAO have issued reports dealing with efforts to control illegal importation [of drugs] and . . . the predominant recurring theme of these reports . . . is the need for greater coordination and cooperation among various enforcement agencies."[67] From a strictly theoretical perspective, it is possible for discrete organizations to pool resources and have few organizational conflicts. As Collins points out, with "pooled activities, especially when the production tasks themselves are highly routine, the problems of control and coordination are minimal."[68] However, the case of border interdiction is anything but routine. In this situation each of the participating agencies realized that the pooling of resources was inherently dangerous for its own organization because such cooperation could lead to reduced autonomy within the law enforcement system: "The more an organization is made up of pooled production activities . . . the lower the power of managers in relation to each other."[69]

Power is a zero sum commodity; the more one adversary has, the less his competitors have. On the surface, information can be shared without one's losing the resource for himself; and in fact the pooling of information would seem to increase the power of each agency by giving each a larger overview of the structure of the smuggling operations. However, organizations are often more interested in perpetuating their own position than effectively carrying out their institutional task. In the case of border law enforcement, information is power and as such becomes a commodity that each agency seems to hoard for its own institutional needs. The overall effectiveness of border interdiction is thus decreased, but narrow ideas of organizational survival seem to be more important to participants than the control of drug smuggling.

CONCLUSIONS

Existential conflict theorists, especially Randall Collins, have focused on a number of organizational issues important to understanding the bureaucratic enforcement of drug laws. Central to all aspects of organizational power is the issue of information control. This central theme has been manifested within four strategic areas in which the drug enforcement bureau has had considerable success.

The first area involved the control of the stage on which emotional displays against drug use were played out. Hamilton Wright initially coordinated the passage of the Harrison Act by generating facts at national and international conferences. This strategy was continued by the FBN with Anslinger's coordination of antidrug legislative hearings at both the state and national levels. Through these efforts, public sentiments against minorities were translated into antidrug legislation, specifically the Marijuana Tax Act. The second organizational strategy, the dissemination of information through the mass media, was reflected in Anslinger's statements on marijuana that were printed in popular magazines and journals. Movies, television coverage, and presentations to schools were all used in the FBN campaigns during the mid-1930s, early 1950s, and late 1960s. Probably the most successful tactic was the control of organizational and legal ambiguities. This third strategy was manifested in the FBN's use of selected Supreme Court decisions when creating organizational guidelines for implementing the Harrison Act. Further, the increased drug use in the early 1950s and late 1960s acted as times of social change in which the bureau attempted to expand its hegemony into areas where its mandate for authority was less than clear. The ambiguous outer edge of bureaucratic authority becomes the target for increased organizational hegemony during times of social upheaval. The final strategy involved the establishment and maintenance of reciprocal interdependence with key government committees. Along with the rise of the FBN as the producers and disseminators of information on the drug issue came a mutual reinforcement system between the bureau and congressional committees. In the case of the drug crisis of the early 1950s and late 1960s, the FBN fit its organizational ideology to the needs of the predominant conspiracy theory on Capitol Hill. Whether charging that the Mafia, communists, or hippies were threatening the nation's moral fiber, both the bureau and Congress supported their counterpart's efforts in solidifying their particular view of reality.

These organizational strategies were built on an information feedback loop established by the Harrison Act. The FBN successfully maintained the dichotomy between minority drug users and the middle-class nonusers, a dichotomy that enabled the overlapping stereotypes of minorities and drug users (both seen as lazy, pleasure seeking, and prone to violence) to go unchallenged. The negative feedback loop was ritually refined and reinforced with the drug crisis of the early 1950s, and the bureau was able to have the legislative penalties for drug use increased. In spite of these successful efforts, some groups, such as musicians and actors, still used drugs. For these artists drug use was a sign of not only rebellion but of an ideology that drugs were a means toward increased awareness and creativity. This pro-drug ideology did not find a significant following until the larger social conditions that originally created the antidrug stereotype were reversed.

Between the passing of the Harrison Act (1914) and the rise of the hippie movement of the late 1960s, the FBN's power went unchallenged. Drug use was the domain of the urban poor, and the bureau successfully employed its strategies to contain it there. Although these minorities, especially the jazz musicians and street users, were somewhat open in their use of drugs, the economic, cultural, and political underpinnings of the negative feedback loop did not change enough to affect the overall structure of drug enforcement. However, this general ebb and flow between stability and minor drug crisis became a hurricane with the rise of a new minority, the hippies. Because of the civil rights movement, economic affluence, and a decline in respect for institutional authority due to the war in Vietnam, the barrier between white and minority cultures began to break down. The economic and cultural factors that originally had generated the negative feedback loop between drug users and nonusers were reversed, and public perception of drugs began to shift. Liberal, educated, middle-class youth came to the urban colonies where drug use became a central factor in the street scenes. The colonies, especially San Francisco's Haight Ashbury, Berkeley's Telegraph Avenue, and New York's Greenwich Village set the stage for a new emotional display. New moral entrepreneurs, now in favor of drugs as a means toward mystical truth, began to be heard in the mass media. The FBN's Harry Anslinger was being replaced by Aldous Huxley, Alan Watts, and Timothy Leary as the new authorities on drugs. The hallucinogenic drugs, LSD, psilocybin, mescaline, and marijuana, became the chemical and idological wedge in the bureau's monopoly on information control.

Faced with a drug crisis of major proportions, the FBN initially responded in its ritualistic manner by calling for expanded government control of drugs and increased penalties against violators. However, it soon became apparent that a major reorganization of the bureau itself would be necessary. After two structural reorganizations, the bureau became the Drug Enforcement Administration, with both domestic and international drug control responsibilities. This wide-ranging mandate came in direct conflict with other government agencies, especially Customs at the international border. Both the DEA and Customs were aware of the importance of information control in the effective apprehension of drug traffickers and in presenting a postive law enforcement image to the larger society. Both agencies have had their differences in strategies, tactics, and results in apprehending smugglers.

3 THE COLD BORDER BUST: ROUTINE APPREHENSION, PROSECUTION, AND PLEA BARGAINING OF DRUG SMUGGLING CASES

Drug smuggling and the law enforcement strategies to control it have had a mercurial quality. Any attempt to impose pressure on smuggling operations along one segment of the American continental border leads to an inevitable fragmentation of smuggling operations in that area and their resurfacing in another location. This has been the character of smuggling operations since the major increase in drug use during the late 1960s, and all evidence indicates that it will continue. Rather than focusing on several geographical areas in which smuggling has surfaced, this analysis is concerned with smuggling along the Mexican-American border, an area in which most of the drugs were smuggled between 1970 and 1978. It was the "Mexican connection" that infused drugs into the American culture during most of the 1970s. It was also the area in which both the DEA and Customs had to develop their individual apprehension strategies and, to some degree, systems of mutual assistance. Public concern over drugs and the development of law enforcement strategies were at their apex when the Mexican connection was the most active area of drug smuggling.

Although smuggling from Mexico was in the limelight for the better part of the 1970s, the years 1978 to 1980 witnessed considerable public and law enforcement concern shifting towards the area along the Gulf Coast. Local, state, and federal law enforcement agencies have given increasing evidence to congressional committees that this area is witnessing a major rise in drug traffic, especially of marijuana and cocaine. The Customs commissioner for the Gulf Coast region indicated this marked increase in his testimony before a congressional subcommittee in 1980:

During fiscal year 1978, our patrols participated in seizures involving approximately 131.4 tons of marijuana. This figure nearly doubled in fiscal 1979 with seizures amounting to 231.6 tons. We feel this is probably as much indicative of the volume of smuggling as it is of our success in meeting the threat.[1]

Although he did not give statistics, the commissioner mentioned a marked increase of cocaine confiscations during this same period. Whether these increases reflect increased drug trafficking, increased law enforcement activities, or some combination of the two, as the commissioner suggested, one can never objectively determine. Irrespective of the ultimate foundation for these increases, the results are the same: increased public titillation of the "drug threat" and the implicit need for effective law enforcement techniques. Although the focus of the interdiction effort in the 1980s will differ from that of the 1970s, the organizational strategies and tactics developed by law enforcement agencies during the 1970s will remain operative. Hence, a close look at the different strategies used by Customs and the DEA along the Mexican-American border will give a clear indication of the organizational structure of antismuggling operations until the next major reorganization plan is deemed necessary. All indications at this time are that the smugglers and law enforcement officials should be settling into a period of stability that could last for as much as a decade or more.

Not only was the majority of law enforcement attention focused on the Mexican-American border during the last decade, but for a number of reasons the most controversial drugs—heroin, cocaine, and marijuana—were infiltrating through that area. There were a number of reasons for this. In the case of marijuana, the warmer and more humid climate of central Mexico produces a potent type of marijuana, which is highly marketable in the United States. By far, the most potent marijuana is grown in Colombia and sells for twice as much as its Mexican counterpart within the American market. Although most of the Colombian marijuana came into the United States through Mexico during the 1970s, it is not as plentiful as Mexican-grown marijuana. During the heaviest period of U.S. involvement in Vietnam, between 1965 and 1973, some marijuana from that area found its way into the American markets. However, the majority of the marijuana bought by American troops in Southeast Asia was smoked there and was not smuggled into the United States.

Cocaine was also essentially a Mexican importation in the 1970s. It is grown in the Andes Mountain regions of Colombia and Peru and processed in the major urban centers of Bogotá, Colombia, and Culiacán, Mexico. From these areas, it was shipped to the United States and distributed to the major metropolitan areas of Los Angeles, Chicago, and New York. With the marked increase in cocaine use in the United States, federal officials have become increasingly intent on controlling this substance. The rise of cocaine on the American market during the period between the revolution in drug use and the mid-1970s is illustrated in the statistics on Customs' confiscations (table 2). There is no way of knowing exactly how much cocaine has been smuggled into this country, but border officials estimate that they are able to apprehend approximately 10 percent of the total traffic. This means that there was approximately 6,000 to 7,000 pounds of cocaine smuggled annually at that time; this number, as expected, increased.

Table 2
CUSTOMS CONFISCATION OF COCAINE, 1965-1975

Year	Coﬁaine Conﬁscated, in Pounds
1965	37
1966	45
1967	40
1968	98
1969	199
1970	227
1971	408
1972	619
1973	592
1974	554
1975	653

Heroin has been the most important drug by far that federal officials have attempted to control. Unlike marijuana or cocaine, it has had several ports of entry into this country, although, like the other drugs, Mexico was the most predominant producer of heroin during the 1970s. Originally the most significant source of illegal heroin was from Turkey. Prior to 1973, the warm, dry climate of Turkey had motivated many of its poorer inhabitants to grow opium poppies for export. After being harvested, the raw opium was shipped to Marseille, France, where it was processed into pure heroin and shipped to distributors in major cities throughout the world, especially New York City. The rapid increase in heroin addiction during the late 1960s motivated both the French and American governments to focus on this line of traffic. By 1974, the "French connection" had been significantly curtailed through the opium ban imposed on the growers in Turkey. In 1973, the U.S. government agreed to buy all of the opium in Turkey and process it for legitimate use in this country. In exchange, the Turkish government agreed to control the illegal cultivation of opium in their country. This agreement significantly eliminated the supply of very pure or so-called white heroin in the American market.

As in the case of marijuana, some heroin found its way into American markets from Southeast Asia due to the presence of American troops in Vietnam. This heroin was grown in an area known as the "golden triangle," which borders eastern Burma and extends across northern Thailand and up into northern Laos. The peasants of this region grew opium as a means of subsistence and sold it to those with the technology to process it and the connections to distribute it internationally. However, with the American withdrawal from Southeast Asia in the early 1970s, this area was no longer a major supplier for American markets for the rest of the decade. The reduction of both the French and Southeast Asian heroin connections gave rise to the "Mexican connection." Federal officials believed that 95 percent of all of the heroin on the American market was smuggled in from Mexico at that time.[2] This heroin, which is grown and processed in Mexico, is termed brown heroin because the processing plants are not as sophisticated and the heroin is a brownish color, as opposed to the pure white of the French-processed, Middle Eastern heroin. Generally, the heroin has been grown in the Mexican state of Durango and has been processed in the city of Culiacán, after which it was shipped into this country.

Although federal officials consider heroin the most important drug to control, their apprehension techniques are designed to control all types of illegal drugs entering into the United States. But the task of apprehending drug smugglers at the international border has become increasingly difficult due to a number of interrelated factors. The most significant of these factors include the increased number of persons crossing the border, the availability of rapid and sophisticated modes of transportation, and the recent increased demand for illicit drugs within the United States. In 1968, approximately 213 million persons crossed the border (205 million persons lived in the United States in that year). This figure increased to approximately 251 million in 1973, indicating an increase of approximately 4 percent for each of the years within that time period. By 1978, the figure had risen to 310 million. One of the major reasons for this increase has been the recent development of various recreational and commercial areas in countries adjacent to the United States. This has been especially true of Mexico, where Americans have found the lax laws and challenging terrain a major inducement for various off-the-road vehicle activities. This has caused numerous problems for border officials, who indicate that "on any given weekend there will be thousands of guys driving their dune buggies and what-not back and forth across the border. Most of them don't even know that they have crossed the international border."[3] This general traffic across the border, both through the official ports of entry and across the hinterland, coupled with the profitability of drug smuggling, has induced many persons of all ages, occupations, and social backgrounds to attempt to add to their income by drug trafficking.

Federal officials[4] informally acknowledge that they have been able to apprehend only an estimated 5 percent of the total smuggling of marijuana and narcotics into the United States.[5] These officials gauge the effectiveness of their efforts by the fluctuation of prices of drugs on the wholesale and retail markets. To the degree that their policies are effective, there will be a scarcity on the market, which will drive up prices. However, as one official stated, "Although a number of different programs have been implemented, the only significant change in prices has been a general and steady increase due to inflation. Our efforts get a percentage off the market, but not enough to significantly alter drug traffic as a whole."[6] Although the government has not been effective in curtailing this activity, it has generated an elaborate system by which it is able to put some pressure on those engaged in the drug traffic.

There has been a considerable disparity between the apprehension procedures used by Customs at the border and those used by the DEA in their attempt to work within both this country and Mexico. Although there was considerable tension between these two organizations over the structuring of information, each agency has had substantial organizational independence to develop its own arrest procedures. The Customs strategy has been to focus exclusively on border interdiction. It has used a complex integration of computerized records, informal detection procedures at the ports of entry, and a roving patrol between border ports. The DEA has emphasized informants who set up the higher-level members of major smuggling rings. Because of these differences in organizational strategies, these two agencies have tended to generate different types of cases. The Customs port of entry arrest usually results in a "cold border bust" in which there are few procedural complications and the case can be processed through the courts in a routine manner. Legal procedural guidelines (especially Fourth Amendment rights to be free from unreasonable search and seizure) are routinely integrated into the practical daily arrest procedures. As such, the prosecution and plea bargaining of these cases takes little time and is handled by the federal courts with relative ease.

The DEA's strategy of setting up busts, however, complicates the arrest and plea-bargaining process, making these much more complex and time-consuming. Essentially the DEA uses plea bargaining to pressure a suspected smuggler (defendant) to set up his connection, who can then be arrested and pressured to set up the next connection up the line. Judicial guidelines relating to the Fourth Amendment and the Fifth Amendment (freedom from self-incrimination) must be integrated into both the arrest and plea-bargaining procedures.

SITUATIONAL AMBIGUITIES IN APPREHENDING SMUGGLERS AT THE INTERNATIONAL BORDER

The manipulation of information in complex and ambiguous situations has been a major theme throughout this book. This theme is also at work in the practical microinteractions between border officials and the smuggling suspect. The situation in which Customs officials have to identify, isolate, and arrest suspected smugglers is problematic for a number of reasons. Most obviously, most of the drugs are concealed by the smugglers, and the official must develop practical techniques for ferreting out this contraband. Of equal importance, the agent must integrate these practical techniques within the general legal procedural guidelines developed by the courts to protect the citizens' constitutional rights. Third, these techniques must be cost-effective in terms of both time and money. In short, the Customs official must effectively develop practical apprehension procedures that fit the smuggler's modus operandi, meet fundamental legal criteria, and effectively fit into allocated organizational resources. By and large, Customs has met these criteria.

The predominant mode of successful detection has been the intensive search of automobiles at the ports of entry. Although it is impossible to determine whether this is the point at which most of the narcotics have been smuggled into the United States, given Customs's focus on this area, it has been the point at which most of the cases are generated that are plea bargained in the federal courts.

The government holds that there are not enough personnel or monetary resources to patrol the entire border adequately; hence the policy has been to concentrate on those areas that act as a funnel for the major part of the civilian traffic crossing the border. For example, there are only four paved roads that cross the border into California, and each has a major checkpoint on the border and another one some distance inland.[7] The theory is that these checkpoints are at the neck of the funnel through which most of the traffic must pass. If the border officials miss a shipment at the port of entry, then there is a possibility of apprehension at the checkpoint farther inland. In order to maximize the detection of possible smugglers with a minimum of detention and inconvenience to persons legitimately crossing the border, government officials have developed an elaborate system of detection using computers, informal typifications, and special legal discretionary powers concerning search and seizure.

The government also uses a contingency of roving patrol officers who are responsible for checking all "suspicious" persons within one hundred miles of the border.[8] In this case they are usually Immigration (INS) rather than Customs agents. Like the officials at the ports of entry, they have developed a system of typifications by which they determine suspiciousness and have a set of procedural rules applicable to the particular circumstances surrounding their work. Given that their work is unique, they are not bound by the full *"probable cause"* requirement, although recent court decisions have indicated that procedural restraints must be adhered to on all official search-and-seizure actions. That is, border officials need less evidence to justify a search of a citizen than police officers working within the United States. However, border officials do not have complete discretionary power and must adhere to a number of recent court rulings.

In terms of procedural due-process constraints on border stops, searches, and seizures, the courts have always differentiated the area around the border from that of the interior of the country. When the Supreme Court made its initial exposition of the Fourth Amendment in 1886, it made special note of the border situation. In *Boyd* vs. *United States*, the Court noted that "the search and seizure of . . . goods liable to duties and concealed to avoid the payment thereof, are totally different from a search for and seizure of . . . a man's private books and papers. The two things differ *toto caelo*."⁹ Here the Court set the stage for the generation of a less stringent set of procedural standards for guiding police discretionary powers at the border. This stance was reiterated and a legitimating basis was generated some forty years later when the Court stated in *Carroll* vs. *United States* (1924) that "travellers may be . . . stopped in crossing the international border because national self-preservation reasonably requires one entering the country to identify himself . . . and his belongings and effects."¹⁰ Hence, the right of a sovereign nation to protect itself provides the basis for justifying the differentiation of due process at the border and procedural constraints within the nation-state itself.

Given these general guidelines generated by the Supreme Court, it has become incumbent upon the Ninth Circuit Court of Appeals, which has jurisdiction over most of the southwestern border area, to explicate the scope of police discretion in more detail. Initially, the circuit court has given broad discretionary powers to U.S. border officials, but in the late 1960s and early 1970s a conscious effort was made to generate guidelines similar to the Supreme Court's classic rulings in *Mapp* v. *Ohio*, *Terry* v. *Ohio*, and *Chimel* v. *California*.[11] In 1936 the circuit court stated in *Landau* v. *United States* that "the search at the border by a government official is of the broadest possible character and any objects seized might be used in evidence."[12] The Court then held in *Alexander* v. *United States* (1966) that "a search that would be held 'reasonable' by a police officer in an ordinary case, is not unreasonable if conducted by a border official."[13] However, in *Thomas* v. *United States* (1967), it held that "a border search and seizure is not completely exempt from the constraints of the Fourth Amendment."[14] The question arises, What are the boundaries of police discretionary powers?

A BRIEF RETURN TO THE EXISTENTIAL-CONFLICT PERSPECTIVE: THE PRACTICAL INTEGRATION OF ORGANIZATIONAL GOALS AND LEGAL CONSTRAINTS IN AN AMBIGUOUS SITUATION

Neither the substantive imperative to apprehend drug smugglers nor the Supreme Court's rulings indicate exactly how agents should operate in the field. The Supreme Court's directives to adhere to the criterion of reasonableness in executing field search and seizure does not explicitly delineate procedural norms. Rather, these rulings imply a set of relatively vague outer markers that are designed to inhibit discretionary abuses. Government agents have more discretionary power at the border than do their counterparts working within the continental United States; nevertheless a border search is not completely free from Fourth Amendment constraints. Here agents are faced with the existential dilemma of how to apply vague procedural guidelines to the highly problematic situation of apprehending clandestine smugglers at the crowded international borders. Given the existential nature of the dilemma, can the existential-conflict perspective shed any light on the situation?

The existential-conflict perspective sees the law as a social construction generated by specific individuals and groups. The same theoretical paradigm can be applied to the law enforcement end of the legal system. At the most general level, the moral entrepreneur, like the law enforcement official, is an intermediary between the law and the public. Just as the moral entrepreneur mediates between public sentiments and the creation of the law, the law enforcement official mediates between the legal mandate and the concrete social situations in which the law is implemented. More specifically, both agents of the legal system must manipulate information within problematic and tense situations in order to meet their particular goals. Whether the agent is attempting to construct public support for antidrug legislation or is attempting to detect suspected smugglers among the masses of individuals who cross the international border, the existential foundation of the situation is the same: the agents must generate information patterns that allow them to define and control ambiguous situations in a manner of their choosing.

Whether the stage is international, national, or one point along the border, the task of the individual is essentially the same. The successful agent controls the information pattern in a way that assures an emotional display that propels events in the desired direction. Wright developed emotional displays within the context of international conferences, while Anslinger worked within the national context of the newly formed FBN. Each controlled information in a manner that facilitated the passage of antidrug legislation. Similarly Customs and the newy formed DEA attempted to generate information patterns that would facilitate their individual organizational goals. Each group made a considerable effort to display a positive image to congressional budgeting committees that would facilitate funding. The same general situation exists between law enforcement officers and suspected smugglers at the microlevel. Officials are faced with an inherently problematic situation in which their major lever of control is the effective structuring of information flow. Central to this process is the manipulation of the situation so that the suspect generates an emotional display that separates him from the ordinary citizen crossing the border. The basic ingredients remain the same: information control, emotional displays, and organizational success.

Although the ingredients are the same, the level of analysis requires an emphasis of the microexistential end of the theoretical paradigm. As Douglas, a leading researcher in the existential-conflict perspective, has remarked:

There is no way of getting at the social meanings from which one either implicitly or explicitly infers the larger patterns [of social order] except through some form of communication with the members of that society or group; and, to be valid and reliable, any such communication with the members presupposes an understanding of their typification, their use of language, their own understanding of what the [situation is in which they are a member].[15]

To understand contemporary apprehension and, ultimately, adjudication procedures, one must turn to the concrete day-to-day use of typifications, language, and their implicit social meanings. Only from this existential base can an accurate understanding of the larger social patterns be achieved.

Over the years, government officials have generated a system of typifications and search-and-seizure techniques that attempts to incorporate the legal standards outlined by the Court. The finite resources available to border officials require that they focus on the ports of entry between Mexico and the United States. At all ports of entry, the search procedure is divided into sections, primary and secondary inspection. As a car or pedestrian approaches the point of inspection, the person is required by law to give his or her name and citizenship and divulge all articles being brought into the United States. At this primary point of inspection, officers are required to filter out those persons whom they believe are most likely to be smuggling contraband and send them to the secondary inspection, which is much more thorough. In order to facilitate this task of filtering suspects at the primary inspection point, border officials have generated a sophisticated set of typifications by which they divert persons to secondary. From a strictly legal perspective, officials do not need any justification to make a thorough inspection of all of a person's belongings and person. The Court stated in *Henderson* v. *United States* (1967) that "the mere fact that a person is crossing the border is sufficient cause for a search. Thus every person crossing our border may be required to disclose the content of his baggage, vehicle ... purse, wallet, or pockets."[16]

Officials can inspect every person crossing the border, but practical considerations—over twenty-eight million persons crossed just one border point at San Ysidro, California, alone in 1973—require discrimination in the search-and-seizure techniques. Hence officials focus on a number of features of the suspect and the particular situation confronting the officer in order to determine which persons should be diverted to secondary inspection. There is wide agreement among police, prosecutors, and defense attorneys that there is no uniform profile of the average drug smuggler, a potential suspect can be of any ethnic, age, sex, and occupational group. There are, however, three essential analytical areas on which border officials focus in order to determine the most fruitful suspect to send to secondary inspection: incongruity in the person's story and/or official papers, suspicious appearance of the car, and the demeanor and presentation of the person. The following example is useful:

Border officials stopped a 1967 Tempest being driven by a male Mexican citizen who was asked to show his driver's license, immigration papers, and car registration. He claimed the car was his, but the names on the registration and the driver's license did not match. He was then told to drive to secondary and was asked to open his trunk. He became nervous and initially placed the key in upside down. The driver was then required to open the hood of the car, where seventy-five kilos of marijuana were found strapped to the inside of the engine compartment.[17]

Although the irregularities of divergent names on the driver's license and car registration, coupled with the suspect's nervousness, were more than enough to legitimate a thorough search of the car and driver, these features of the situation also act as indexes of a larger smuggling picture. Immigration and customs officials have a system of typifications that not only determines which persons are likely suspects but also typifies the location of the suspect within the overall structure of drug traffic.

In this example, the case represents a "typical mule" who is hired by a trafficker or a large dealer in Mexico to transport the contraband across the border. Typically, persons engaged in growing and transporting marijuana from the interior of Mexico to the border will attempt to get such a person to take the contraband across the border. Given the large labor pool of unemployed and marginally employed Mexican nationals and Mexican-Americans, it is easy for a dealer to hire a mule. Usually, the mule is given from $100 to $500 to drive the car a few hundred yards from a parking lot, in say Tijuana, to a lot just inside San Ysidro. Thus, the dealer will structure the transportation operation such that the point of most risk (the border crossing) will be taken by a person who is not connected or is only marginally connected with the overall operation. In one case, the mule was paid $250, but the gross profit on the seventy-five kilograms would have been approximately $50,000 by the time that the marijuana was sold.

In cases involving mules, an important element in a prosecution concerns the necessity of proving both knowledge and control over the contraband. The border officials must focus on the situation in such a way as to glean indications that the driver was aware of the contraband in the vehicle. This is usually accomplished by noting the suspect's emotional reactions to the inspector's probe into certain parts of the car. If the suspect makes specific and articulable types of errors (such as placing the key in the trunk lock upside down) and these mistakes can be considered signs of nervousness, then a strong case can be made against the driver. If the driver of the car is also the licensed owner of the car, this is prima facie evidence of both knowledge and control. Most mules, however, do not own the car they drive across, and the border official must generate evidence to prove the necessary legal connection between the driver and the contraband.

Another example illustrates the typification process used by border officials to determine possible smugglers in terms of the cars driven across the border:

A 1970 Ford was observed approaching the checkpoint and the border officer noticed that there seemed to have been some body work done on one of the fender panels. The car had numerous scratches all over it, except along this one fender panel. The official tapped the fender and it sounded solid [a lower pitched tap]. The car was ordered to secondary, where the removal of the fender revealed one hundred and twenty-five kilos of marijuana.[18]

The focusing on cars is structured according to the same incongruity procedure involved in checking stories and official papers; however, this aspect of the border search is facilitated by a computer. Each of the checkpoints has a computer with an input and output display at both the primary and secondary inspection points. As each car drives toward the primary inspection point, the officer feeds in the car's license plate and, in return, a light goes on indicating "hit" or "OK." If the light indicates "hit," it means that there is information within the computer relating this car with some drug problem. All known addicts, dealers, and users of drugs who own cars have had their license number fed into the computer. Any information from informants in Mexico or the United States and the records of all persons arrested and/or convicted of drug offenses are coded according to names and/or license numbers. Hence, when the primary inspection point indicates "hit," the driver is sent directly to secondary, at which time the computer display at secondary reveals the specific information relating to that car.

The places in which contraband can be hidden in an automobile are limited only by the smuggler's imagination. The small size of narcotics (heroin, cocaine, and opium) and pills (barbiturates and amphetamines of various kinds) allows for more diverse forms of concealment than the bulky marijuana, which is usually hidden in the paneling or spare tire of a car or is stacked in the trunk or engine compartment. Because of the size and the tendency for large amounts of marijuana to give off a strong odor, especially on hot days, inspection efforts are usually successful once a car with large amounts of marijuana has been diverted to secondary inspection.

The narcotics, on the other hand, require more effort on the part of border officials for successful detection. Narcotics have been found in hollowed-out crutches, casts on broken legs, the brake drums of cars, and other small and concealed areas of a car. Given these differences, fewer arrests are made for narcotics and pills than for marijuana. When an arrest is made for substances in this latter category, it is usually due to the demeanor of the suspect rather than an incongruity concerning the car.[19] Generally most border officials rely primarily on the demeanor and presentation of the suspect as the major criterion for requiring a secondary inspection.

In terms of demeanor, the most common and pervasive focus by border officials is on the various cues that indicate nervousness. As the driver approaches, officials check the person's knuckles to see if they are pale from gripping the steering wheel too tightly, if there is any perspiration around the hairline due to tension, if the vein in the neck is palpitating rapidly, the pace and intensity of the person's respiration, and any shaking of parts of the body. Nervous persons often have difficulty in various manual operations, such as opening a door, handing papers to an officer, and talking. Thus these operations are closely scrutinized and act as objective indexes of nervousness that are admissible in court.

The primary checkpoint official gives the secondary official a brief statement as to why an individual is diverted to secondary. At secondary, the officials have the legal discretion to expand the search throughout the car until they are satisfied that there is no contraband. Because the suspect's nervousness is a primary criterion for the search, the secondary officer often monitors the suspect's demeanor while searching the car. If the suspect becomes more nervous as the officer works, the officer will intensify his search in that area. The smaller size of heroin and pills gives rise to a number of legal and practical considerations. The law gives border officials almost complete discretionary powers to search and seize any contraband among the possessions of any person crossing the international border. Whether an officer will thoroughly search a person's car is a practical question involving time available, the number of persons on shift, and the number of persons crossing the border. There are few legal constraints involved in investigations limited to the property and/or patdown of the person. Small amounts of narcotics, however, can be hidden in body cavities, highly private areas where police discretionary powers have been curtailed in searches. The following case exemplifies the problems and procedures involved in detecting narcotics on the person's body:

A white female in her late teens approached the border official checking pedestrians crossing the border at the San Ysidro checkpoint. The officer noticed the girl was shaking and asked her to hold out her hands, palms down, and noted that her hands were shaking severely. When asked why she was nervous, she responded, "I came down to Tijuana with my boyfriend to go to some bars, but I didn't like it down there. My boyfriend is still down there, but I'm going home." The officer diverted her to secondary inspection.

In secondary, the girl was asked to empty her pockets, her purse, and roll up her sleeves. In her purse officials found two plane tickets to Los Angeles and the usual articles of feminine grooming. When asked about the tickets, she indicated that she and her boyfriend had flown down to Tijuana for the weekend and that she was going to fly back. The official asked how her boyfriend was going to fly back since she had both of the tickets. At this point the suspect became visibly more nervous (increased intensity and rapidity of breathing and shaking). Finally, a check of the suspect's arms revealed "track marks" of a possible heroin addict.

The suspect was then taken into the next room by a female official and was given a "strip search" in which her clothing was removed and a visual examination of her body was conducted. The suspect was asked to spread her feet and bend over so that the official could check the genital area for indications that a foreign object might be in the anus or vagina. The suspect spread her feet about a foot and bent over, however, there was no overt indication of any foreign object. However, the official did note that the "suspect's buttock was quivering as if she was trying to hold something in." The suspect was allowed to dress and the female officer relayed her findings to her supervisor. The latter then called the U.S. Attorney's Office for permission to conduct a "full body cavity search", received permission and had the female official conduct such a search.

The search consisted of requiring the suspect to disrobe, bend over and manually part the opening of her anus and vagina for the inspection by the official with a flashlight. At that time the official noticed a "white foreign substance" in her vagina. The official then informed the suspect that either she could remove the object herself or the officials would take her to a licensed physician to have it removed. The suspect removed the object and it was found to be a condom containing fifty grams of heroin.[20]

This example deals with search-and-seizure issues that have recently become the focus of Ninth Circuit Court decisions concerning highly personal areas of one's body. Prior to the advent of the Warren Court's decisions concerning procedural due process (1962–1968), the Ninth Circuit Court tended to take border search-and-seizure cases on a case-by-case basis, making no overt attempt to generate specific guidelines for search-and-seizure procedures. Because the Supreme Court had always given border officials discretion in the search of personal property at the border, the Ninth Circuit Court was reluctant to make any absolute restrictions concerning such searches. Only the most flagrant intrusions in terms of body cavity searches were ruled unreasonable by the southern California court. However, with the Warren Court's attempt to set specific guidelines for search-and-seizure procedures in *Terry, Mapp,* and *Chimel,* the circuit court had a basis on which to legitimate specific guidelines at their local border areas. With the trend set by the Warren Court, civil libertarian attorneys began to appeal various cases that involved possible abuse of police discretionary powers at the border.

There was no doubt in the minds of either the police or the liberal attorneys that the police needed something less than full probable cause to search and seize articles at the border, but there was strong feeling that some criterion, less than probable cause, should be generated to legitimate searches into a person's private areas. The major case in this area was *Henderson* v. *United States* (1967). This decision outlined four criteria considered effective in governing police discretionary powers. These criteria include "mere suspicion," "founded suspicion," "clear indication," and finally the full "probable cause." The criterion of "mere suspicion" is the least constraining and includes any belief that the officer may have that a person is violating the law. As a practical matter, this is more a descriptive term indicating that the officer simply decided to invoke his discretionary powers to search a person rather than an objective criterion to be met prior to any search. When mere suspicion exists, it justifies only a search of the individual's personal belongings and a limited search of the person's body—such as an exterior patdown and an inspection of pockets. Here the complete search of a person's automobile is permissible, and, hence, the discovery of large quantities of marijuana at the port of entry is usually made under such criteria. Given the limited and possibly nonexistent criteria of such a search, these cases seldom have search-and-seizure issues promoted as a defense. However, in the case of narcotics that are hidden on the suspect's private person, the more stringent criteria of founded suspicion and clear indication are often issues contested within the plea-bargaining negotiations.

The use of a strip search, in which the suspect disrobes for a visual inspection of the body, must be based on a real or founded suspicion. This verbal formula requires the official to be able to articulate specific features of the situation that lead him or her to suspect the person of hiding contraband. This criterion is similar to those outlined in *Terry*, in that the officer must have observable and articulable criteria, not just a hunch or suspicion, to justify a search. In the example case, the extreme nervousness of the suspect, as indicated by the shaking hands, the incongruity of flying to Tijuana simply to go to some bars and then leaving her boyfriend stranded with no ticket home, and the track marks indicating possible narcotic addiction constituted a solid basis for founded suspicion. In this case the officers had specific criteria that they could elucidate that founded their suspicion that the person might be harboring narcotics. Probably the most significant indicator was the track marks. In this area officials have attempted to increase the basis for their search by determining the age of the track marks. If they are fairly recent, then the decision to search is indisputable. However, if the track marks are bluish and are turning brown or are brown, then they are several weeks and possibly months old.[21] In these cases, the prosecution's case can become weakened through the defense's indicating a discriminatory policy against possible ex-addicts on the part of the officials. There is justification for suspecting anyone with indications of having used narcotics, but the closer the connection between the use of drugs and the time one crosses the border, the stronger the case. In the example case, both the prosecution and the defense agreed that the defendant's track marks were recent and that a strip search was justified.

Although searching a suspect is often a routine process, there has been some concern recently over the next step, the body cavity search. It is common for persons to differentiate degrees of privacy in terms of the exterior skin as opposed to the internal organs of one's body. Given the strong norms surrounding one's right to privacy of sexual and related organs, the structuring of police discretion relative to the extraction of articles thought to be inside a person has been a point of legal controversy. The first major Supreme Court decision outlining the parameters of this area was the drinking driver case of *Schmerber* v. *California* (1968). In this case, the Court ruled it legitimate for the police to require a registered doctor or nurse to remove a sample of blood from a person suspected of drunken driving. Such a removal is justified in those situations in which the officer has a clear indication that the person was under the influence of alcohol. In this case, Schmerber had alcohol on his breath and was extremely uncoordinated in his speech and physical movements. Thus, there were specific empirical indicators that pointed directly to possible intoxication, a significant distinction from the more general empirical indicators that support a founded suspicion criterion. A founded suspicion may be justified by a number of general features of the suspect or the situation (nervousness, incongruity of official papers, or incongruous accounts of one's behavior or effects); however, none of these indicators points directly to the possibility of smuggling contraband. On the contrary, there may be any number of reasons for explaining these general incongruities. On the other hand, the smell of alcohol and a lack of coordination point directly to intoxication, and the track marks (especially if recent) point directly to narcotics use. Hence, the clear indication criterion is a much closer nexus between a specific indicator and a specific legal violation than the founded suspicion.

This verbal formula was applied to narcotics search and seizures at the border by the Ninth Circuit Court in *Henderson* v. *United States* (1967). As a practical matter, "clear indication" refers to any physical object that points directly to contraband residing in a specific part of the body. The most common clear indications are strings protruding from the anal or vaginal cavity, indicating easier access to an object in that cavity; Vaseline or other lubricants around the cavity, indicating easier placement of a foreign object; and actual protruding of a foreign object. In one case, none of these indicators were present and the sole basis for the body cavity search was the subjective interpretation of "tight buttocks" as an indication of "attempting to hide something" on the part of the officer. Had any of the physical clear indications been present, there would have been no basis for the defensc's attempt to suppress evidence. However, the invoking of the subjective criterion as the clear indication required the court to review the totality of the facts in determining the legitimacy of the search. In this case, the fact that the defendant had track marks, generated an account that was internally inconsistent, was nervous, and appeared to be hiding something was enough to justify the full search.

A number of generalizations can be made about the typifications, legal restraints, and practical procedures for controlling situations at ports of entry. Officials tend to typify suspects in terms of the amount of drugs found in their possession and from that extrapolate the defendant's relation to the organized smuggling operation. Essentially the predominant type of smuggler found at the border is the small-time dealer-user of narcotics and the marijuana mule. These are the persons who actually take the risk of carrying the contraband through the most heavily inspected points along the border. The mule carries the burden of the risk at the border, while the larger dealer grows and ships the contraband to the border and/or distributes it once it is inside the United States. The small-time dealer-user, on the other hand, usually takes only a few kilograms of marijuana and/or a few ounces of narcotics across the border to satisfy his personal habit and/or distribute to a few other users for extra money. Neither of these types of smugglers is making large percentages of the profit available in the trafficking of drugs, and few have strong connections with larger dealers.

Border officials have generated a practical apprehension system that incorporates the fundamental legal constraints outlined by the courts with the situational resources inherent within the border situation. Given that the border situation is inherently problematic and tension inducing, border officials have used the emotional displays of the suspected smugglers as a tool for their apprehension. Not only do specific forms of incongruity in one's papers and one's behavior isolate potential suspects, but each also acts as a guide for leading the inspector to the contraband. Through practical field investigations, officers have generated informal procedures through which these displays identify suspects, tie the suspect to the contraband, and become the legal foundation for the subsequent plea bargaining.

Once the smuggler gives the border official cause to single him out for further inspection at secondary, the likelihood of detecting marijuana is very high and the detection of narcotics and pills is reasonably high. If drugs are found in the automobile or among other possessions of the suspect, no search-and-seizure issues can undermine the prosecution of the case. However, drugs hidden in the body cavity may be an issue for attempts by the defense to suppress evidence, but on the whole, most members of the law enforcement agency and the courts see busts at the port of entry as "cold border busts." That is, if the officers have attempted to fulfill those few procedural restraints imposed on them by the courts, there is little possibility of an acquittal through the suppression of illegally seized evidence.

The Roving Patrol

Of the three forms of apprehending drug smugglers—port of entry inspections, roving patrol inspections, and informants—the first two methods are the most closely related in method and procedure. The border patrol (Customs and Immigration) is divided into those working the "still watch" at the ports of entry and those responsible for a "roving patrol" of the hundreds of miles between the ports of entry. Although the same members of the border patrol generate arrests in both areas by being circulated or rotated between these areas every six or eight months, there are significant differences in the quality of cases produced by these two forms of patrol. This is due primarily to the circumstances surrounding the different methods of patrol, procedural rules governing the areas patrolled, and the organizational checks on actual apprehension procedures used by personnel in the field.

From a strictly legal perspective, the roving patrol has a number of problems concerning the scope of their discretionary powers that are not incumbent upon those working the still watch. The roving patrol must actually observe the suspect crossing the border in order to invoke legitimately the wide discretionary powers of a border search. If a person is observed crossing the border, the officer may elect to follow the vehicle and stop and search the car some distance from the border under the notion of an extended border search. As one border official noted, "Since most of the guys driving across the border are just mules, it is often wise to follow the car to wherever he is going to make his connection or stash the stuff. This way we nab the whole bunch and there aren't any search and seizure complications under an extended border search."[22] This means that an officer can stop, search, and arrest persons with the same discretionary powers he has at the port of entry, provided that he observes the car crossing the border.

As a practical matter, however, many persons and/or vehicles are sighted near the border, but there is no prima facie evidence that they have actually crossed it. Under these circumstances the typification process and legal restraints relating to search and seizure have become complex and often confusing. According to statute, "An immigration official may search any vehicle for aliens within a reasonable distance from any external boundary of the United States for the purpose of patrolling the border to prevent illegal entry of aliens into the United States."[23] In 1967, the Congress defined "reasonable distance" as extending up to one hundred air miles from the border.[24] Thus, within the jurisdiction of one hundred miles, the border patrol was relatively free in their discretionary powers to stop, search, and arrest persons suspected of being or aiding the illegal entry of aliens. This, in turn, led to many drug arrests free of search and seizure issues. A border official described it this way: "A large number, perhaps half or so, of our arrests were due to a patrolman seeing a car out in the middle of nowhere coming from the border. Invariably the car was full of Mexicans and was weighted down in the back. The officer would stop the car and check the trunk and find a whole stash of marijuana."[25] The discovery of drugs while checking for alien smuggling was procedurally proper conduct.

The possible and actual abuse of such power seriously threatened the legitimate members of the Mexican-American community on the U.S. side of the border, as well as legally entering aliens who reside near the border. Members of these groups organized and pressured the government to set stricter criteria for border stops and searches. In an attempt to create a solution to this potentially volatile problem, the Ninth Circuit Court ruled that all police-citizen contact that did not fit the strict criterion of a border and/or extended border search were to be conducted under the probable cause criterion of the Fourth Amendment. This decision, *Almeida-Sanchez* v. *United States* (1973), required that all of the Fourth Amendment requirements and their progeny (*Terry, Mapp,* and *Chimel*) strictly limit border searches and seizures. Further, the decision explicitly requires that the officer prove that his stop was founded (under *Terry*) by proving that it could not be interpreted as an arbitrary decision and, hence, a form of racial harassment.

From the perspective of law enforcement officers, the *Sanchez* restrictions seriously undercut their ability to apprehend both alien smuggling and drug traffic offenders. One U.S. attorney has said:

Prior to *Sanchez* many of our cases involved the stopping of vehicles driven by persons of Mexican descent who were seen on a dirt road coming from the border. When asked for ID, many would have false papers or the driver would not have the proper papers. The border patrol could still require the driver to open the trunk and search the car. However, now if the driver has the proper papers and there is nothing to give the officer probable cause to suspect aliens and/or drugs, there is nothing we can do to catch them.[26]

Although the legal restraints on police discretionary powers may undercut their ability to apprehend suspected smugglers, they have generated a number of techniques to fulfill their police function. Given the vast areas that must be covered and the relatively small force used, the border patrol has attempted to focus its efforts in terms of those areas that it believes are used most by smugglers.

They have both ground and air patrol vehicles used to follow vehicles that have been identified by informants as shipping contraband at a specific time and place. To focus resources in the most productive areas, officials attempt to determine those areas most used by smugglers through a number of tactics. Initially, officials concentrate their efforts in those areas where the topography is most conducive to travel. In areas where mountains or rivers make travel difficult or impossible, the area is randomly checked by either plane or vehicle. In areas where travel, especially by automobile, is possible, the roads are "dragged" in order to determine the amount of traffic that passes over them. Throughout much of the open border area between the different checkpoints, there are numerous dirt roads crossing the border. In order to determine the amount of traffic and possible smuggling on these roads, border officials will clean the tire tracks off the road periodically by dragging an object (usually a piece of cyclone fence) behind an automobile. In this manner, the road becomes smooth, and recent tire tracks can be discerned. By periodic checking of these roads, officials are able to determine the amount of traffic on each road, the area in which the cars entered and left the roads, and, hence, the most fruitful areas to patrol. Any car seen near the border can be traced by its tire marks, indicating whether it came from a direction along the border. If the officer can verify that there were tire tracks indicating the car had crossed the border, he can search the car with less than probable cause.

Finally, official efforts to apprehend persons using sophisticated equipment, such as private planes and boats, are very constrained. For example, there are only two radar stations along the 140-mile border between Mexico and California. These FAA radar stations are concerned with directing high-flying commercial and military aircraft, not with low-flying private aircraft. Further, radar is able to cover an area of only 30 to 50 miles at very low altitudes (five hundred feet or less), and so most smugglers are able to fly under the radar net. Thus, both technical and organizational limitations give a relatively free hand to smugglers with the financial resources to fly or ship cargo across the border.

On the whole, border officials must concentrate their efforts on areas known to be common points of drug traffic. These points are determined by geographical structures, knowledge of vehicle travel over various roads, and information on specific shipments gleaned from informants. Once resources have been concentrated in an area, there are a number of indexes used by officials to gain the required probable cause to search vehicles. One common situation is illustrated in this example:

> A vehicle patrolman noticed the suspect's car driving north on a dirt road a few miles north of the international border. As the car passed, the officer noticed weeds stuck under the door panel indicating that the car may have been driven off of the road. Although the two cars were the only ones within the immediate area, the driver passed and seemed to avoid acknowledging the existence of the officer's jeep [would not look in the direction of the officer].
>
> The officer stopped the car and asked the driver for his driver's license, which was rendered and indicated the driver was a legal Mexican immigrant. At that point the officer queried the driver as to his reason for being in the area. The driver seemed very nervous, and became more nervous when asked about the content of the trunk and engine compartment. At that point the officer began to smell the odor of bulk marijuana and required the driver to open the trunk where one hundred kilos of marijuana were found.[27]

Like all other border officials, the roving patrol focuses its attention on certain features of the situation and attempts to derive indexes that will legitimate further investigation. In the case here, the officer focused on aspects of the car that may indicate that the car had crossed the border: the direction in which the car was traveling, weeds stuck under the door panels indicating possible off-the-road travel, and the demeanor of the driver. The location of the car and the general features of the situation provided the basis for a stop and brief questioning under the ruling of *Terry*. The officer, however, had no probable cause to believe that the car actually crossed the border and, hence, would be subject to an extended border search, or that the occupants had actually engaged in illegal activity and could be searched under the Fourth Amendment provisions. Under these circumstances the officer was required to develop probable cause while questioning the driver, or he had to release the driver within a reasonable time under *Lingo* v. *California* (1969).

This process of developing grounds for a further search is similar to the methods used by officers at the port of entry. The driver is required to show proper identification, which is scrutinized for possible incongruities and defects, the car is noted for possible cues that drugs may be concealed within, and the demeanor of the driver is observed and his reactions are noted. In this case, the sun and the large amount of marijuana created an odor detectable by the officer, which was probable cause to search the car.

Had the officer not been able to detect the contraband by smell, the correct license and immigration papers presented by the driver would require the officer to improvise other methods of generating probable cause. The driver's nervousness was not enough to provide probable cause unless the officer could prove that the nervousness was actually due to illegal activity—a nexus that most members of the court feel is practically impossible to provide. For this reason, most officers tend to focus on the interior of the car to see if there is any contraband visible from where they stand outside the car. Often an officer will ask the driver if he can search the car; sometimes a nervous and/or inexperienced mule will give such permission. In this case, all evidence is admissible in court. If the officer feels strongly that there is contraband in the car but is not able to generate the necessary probable cause, he can call for another car and/or plane to follow the car secretly to its destination. Often the activity at the destination (such as several people carrying large bags from the car into the house) will provide the necessary probable cause.

The possibilities of abuse of police discretionary powers under these circumstances are always present and of concern to the courts. As one member of the bench said:

Some of these cases you know the arresting officer did not follow the fine line of procedural due process. They get some guy out in the middle of the desert and they want to know what he has in the trunk, they make him open it. If the defense attempts to suppress the evidence, they just say that they smelled the stuff, the driver gave his permission to search the car, or some such story. It's the cop's word against the driver's and no one else is out there. The fact that they did find the stuff is at least a psychological point against anyone believing the driver's story.[28]

It is impossible to know exactly how closely border officials follow the procedural requirement when they are not under direct supervision. Officials at the port of entry are under close supervision from their law enforcement supervisors, however, and routinely contact a U.S. attorney prior to conducting body cavity searches; thus port of entry searches are usually conducted within constitutional limits. However, the roving patrol is not under direct supervision, and there are practical problems in attempts to gain either a search warrant or probable cause out in the field. Thus, the likelihood that officers will follow their personal hunches and fabricate a story to fulfill legal requirements is greater under these circumstances.

In sum, the situational contingencies surrounding port of entry, as opposed to roving patrol, cases significantly affect the quality of the case when it is plea bargained. At the ports of entry, border officials actually observe suspects crossing the border, which significantly increases their discretionary powers. This, coupled with the courts' specific guidelines dealing with body cavity searches, makes these searches relatively routine. The government officials have generated practical means of computerizing information, typifying suspects, and integrating these typifications into the procedural guidelines developed by the courts. In short, the agents have developed a practical means of controlling information within the problematic situation of border searches. This, in turn, creates the "cold border bust" in which only body cavity searches and, in rare instances, the strip search are complicated with Fourth Amendment issues when adjudicated.

In the case of the roving patrol, however, their distance from on-the-spot supervision, the full procedural restraint incumbent upon most of their arrests, and the lack of other witnesses make adherence to procedural due process more problematic. Unless the suspect is observed actually crossing the border, the *Terry* criterion must be met for the stop and search; border officials must invoke the same general tactics that are found at the port of entry searches. The increased legal constraint, coupled with the inherent tension between police and the suspected smuggler, produces a much more ambiguous case, however. When the ability to control information is both legally and practically in the hands of the law enforcement agents, the cases are dealt with in a routine manner. But in those areas between border ports of entry, where agents have significantly less control, the resulting arrests are more problematic and, hence, weaker when plea bargained.

PLEA BARGAINING NARCOTICS CASES

The U.S. Attorney's Office for the Ninth Circuit Court was under a significant amount of pressure to prosecute the numerous cases generated by the increased use of drugs during the late 1960s. Hence, there was a move to increase the number of deputy attorneys from four in 1968 to thirty-three in 1978 and to organize the office along more bureaucratic lines.

There are a number of important differences in the structure of the U.S. Attorney's Office as compared to the large bureaucratic systems common in most district attorney's offices found in major metropolitan areas. Unlike these larger offices, the U.S. Attorney's Office is not as bureaucratic in terms of specific divisions of labor or hierarchical decision making. Whereas the district attorney's offices are often divided into specialized committees, the federal prosecutors are less constrained by formal procedures in the assignment of particular kinds of cases to the various deputies and the actual prosecution of these cases.

Cases are processed through two separate stages. The case initially is sent from the border official to the "complaint department" where an initial evaluation and appropriate charges are determined, and from there the case is sent to the particular U.S. deputy attorney who will be responsible for the plea bargaining and/or trial. Hence, unlike the district attorney's office, which may pass a single case through three or four different attorneys (for example, presiding deputy, trial deputy, settings and motion deputy, and back to the trial deputy), the federal cases are processed primarily by the initial complaint deputy doing the initial charging; all of the actual plea bargaining is done by one trial deputy.

Members of the U.S. Attorney's Office are quick to mention the advantages of such a system. First, the quality of the prosecution is seen to be enhanced by having one person responsible for the case throughout its adjudication. Given the complexities of some search-and-seizure issues, the necessity of working closely with arresting and investigating officers in presenting a case to the court, and the possibility of drawn-out plea-bargaining negotiations, it is important that one attorney be responsible for the entire process and thus act as a central coordinator of this process and be in a strong position to defend the interests of the state. If the case is shifted between longitudinally specialized attorneys, the continuity and sophistication of the prosecution's case may be undermined.

Further, prosecutors argue that plea bargaining and a speedy conclusion of cases is advanced by this procedure. By having one attorney prosecute the case throughout the adjudication process, the defense attorney will not be tempted to hold out a final plea in hopes of plea bargaining with a more lenient prosecutor at a later stage of the proceedings. At the state level, in contrast, defense attorneys, even in cases in which all of the issues can be resolved in a routine manner, would often proscrastinate in entering a plea in hopes of getting a better bargain later. But, on the federal level this problem is negligible, and the federal attorneys feel that cases are processed much more efficiently.

Finally, the individuated nature of the U.S. Attorney's Office tends to generate more well-rounded attorneys and indirectly produces better defense attorneys. Those deputy attorneys who are planning to work for the federal prosecutor for a limited amount of time and then go into private practice are given a broader scope of experience in both the variety of cases handled and the various stages at which a case is handled, experience that facilitates their ability to draw on a wide range of different cases and gives them insight into the prosecution's perspective on various types of cases—knowledge that will be beneficial in their capacity as defense attorney. These attorneys will have first-hand knowledge of the relative importance of various crimes in the eyes of the prosecution, as well as the probable appropriate plea bargain for a given set of circumstances.

Concomitant with these perceived advantages are a number of disadvantages that affect the quality of prosecuting drug cases. The most important is the probability that similar cases will not be treated similarly. As one deputy attorney noted, "I have almost complete discretion in plea bargaining my cases as long as they stay within reason; there are no formal policies. However, most attorneys recognize that there is a general informal charging policy and I think most of us stick to it."[29] This relatively loose structure may in fact function as well as the formal structures that exist on the state level, especially in the district attorney's office, but it does not have the normal hierarchical checking policies that control state prosecutors. Thus, uniformity of prosecution at the federal level is somewhat more problematic.

Although there is less overt bureaucratic control in the U.S. Attorney's Office, there are informal modes of structuring the flow of cases and generating typifications concerning plea bargaining. More specifically, the initial charging takes place in the "complaint department," which is made up of three attorneys who determine whether a case is strong enough to prosecute, the appropriate initial charge, and the best trial attorney to prosecute the case. Each attorney who works for the federal prosecutor is given an internship in the complaint department, where each is socialized into the informal procedures and typifications used in charging and plea bargaining cases. This is the most routine and bureaucratic stage of the proceedings, with one senior attorney responsible for guiding the initial charges, and the decision about appropriate charges being determined by a standard system of typifications.

Initial Charging Policies

After an arrest, the law enforcement agency writes an arrest report (termed "information" at the federal level) and sends it to the complaint department. The attorney first looks at the amount of drugs involved and the number of prior arrests of the defendant. From these two indexes, the complaint department attorney is able to apply, almost mechanically, a given charge to the cases processed through the office. In the cases involving marijuana, if the defendant has no known prior record and the amount is seen to be a small amount for personal use, then the defendant usually will be charged with a misdemeanor possession violation. More specifically, a person found to have a few lids (that is, up to four lids [five to six ounce bags] on his person is charged with "possession of a controlled substance," a charge having a maximum penalty of one year in jail and up to a $5,000 fine.[30]

The more severe felony options open to the complaint attorney for use in initial charging include possession with intent to distribute[31] and illegal importation of a controlled substance.[32] Both have harsher penalties. Thus, if the defendant is found to be in the possession of larger amounts of marijuana, indicating to the prosecutor that he has intentions of selling the drugs, two felony and one lesser included misdemeanor charge may be applied to that single illegal act.[33] In most cases, the complaint attorney will apply all three charges to persons thought to be intending to sell the drug upon entering the United States. A person caught with ten kilograms at the port of entry will be charged with possession, possession with intent to distribute, and illegal importation of a controlled substance. Each of the felony charges could bring as much as fifteen years in prison and up to a $25,000 fine. Thus, a person convicted on all charges and given the maximum sentence could spend thirty-one years in prison and pay $55,000 in fines.

A second level of charging involves defendants who have been caught conspiring with others in the smuggling of drugs. If a person is caught with another person in the car or there is information of other persons being active in the importation of a sizable amount of marijuana, the complaint department official will add two new charges to the indictment.[34] The individual will be charged with the crimes of possession, possession with intent to distribute, and illegal importation of a controlled substance, plus conspiracy to possess a controlled substance with intent to distribute[35] and conspiracy to import a controlled substance illegally.[36] Thus, more than one person indicted in a given act enables the prosecutor to generate five separate counts with a possible total penalty of a $105,000 fine and sixty-one years in jail.

A number of severe penalties are available to the prosecution in determining the appropriate charge for a given drug violation. Most federal prosecutors agree that the U.S. Congress has generated laws that are too severe if they were to be applied directly to and in toto to each case that is processed through the courts. As one prosecutor mentioned:

The laws governing drug abuse are often too harsh when taken on face value. Thus, from a prosecutor's perspective it is beneficial to have numerous harsh laws to apply to any given case, for this increases our power in the plea bargaining situation. But the Congress is removed from actual and practical processes of apprehending and adjudicating drug offenders and, too, they are under the constantly shifting pressure of public opinion that is often overly punitive due to a blown-up view of drug abuse. Given these forces it is not surprising that drug laws are constantly shifting and are often an over-reaction in terms of punitive sanctions. It is for this reason that the federal prosecutor attempts to fit the law to the particular case in an equitable manner, to temper the law in the interest of justice.[37]

There is a significant amount of agreement among defense attorneys that this is representative of the policy of the U.S. Attorney's Office. Unlike the state prosecutor, who will attempt to prosecute most drug cases to the limit, in many cases the federal prosecutor is willing to make an initial charge less than the maximum and plea bargain most cases involving no prior record on the part of the defendant.[38]

Thus, it is the policy of the complaint department to charge all persons with indictments of possession of a kilogram or less of marijuana with a misdemeanor and place the full felony possession and conspiracy charges as they apply. The full charging of persons thought to be involved in the commercial transaction of drugs is a means of ensuring strength in the prosecutor's case, but the tendency to drop most of these charges readily in the plea-bargaining situation is substantial. This indicates that the basis for the decision to apply a particular charge to a particular case rests with an attempt to differentiate cases according to whether the defendant is a dealer or a user of drugs and to increase the initial charge on the former in order to ensure a strong case for the plea-bargaining situation. Similarly, the lesser charging of the user of marijuana makes it unlikely that he will use up court resources by actually going to trial. Further, a reduction of the charge and sentence to a very nominal fine and / or suspension of jail is seen to be more in line from an initial charge of a misdemeanor. Hence, even though it is possible for the prosecution to charge a person with a felony for less than a kilogram of marijuana, this policy is eschewed in order to focus resources on the larger dealer-smuggler and to enable substantial reductions, which may be negotiated while plea bargaining, to seem more rational.

In the case of heroin and cocaine the complaint department routinely charges the individual with the full number of counts available because of a number of factors that relate specifically to hard narcotics: the possibility of addiction on the part of the smuggler, the more severe social damage done by narcotics, and the difficulty in apprehending small amounts of narcotics at the border. Also, the levying of all relevant charges increases the state's leverage when requiring that an addict-smuggler join a withdrawal program as one of the conditions of the settlement. Usually addicts do not want to quit their habit and the high charges made by the complaint department make it more likely that the addict will agree to such a program. Finally, both because of public sentiment and prosecutor's understanding of the social problems generated by narcotics addiction, such as smuggling and secondary crime, there is an emphasis on making the initial charges the fullest possible under the law. Hence, persons apprehended with a small amount for personal use are charged with felony possession with intent to distribute, and persons who have interacted with someone during the transaction are given the appropriate conspiracy charges in conjunction with either of the other two base charges.

On the whole, the complaint department serves a number of functions for controlling potential ambiguities that may arise within the plea-bargaining process. First, it makes a basic dichotomy between those cases to be pursued seriously and those that will be significantly reduced and/or dismissed. Second, the charging policy of the prosecution gives the trial deputy a number of charges from which to develop a strong bargaining position. Finally, the complaint department acts as a clearinghouse through which cases are distributed to the various trial attorneys. Here again, the discretionary power of the complaint department is guided by the need to maximize the state's control of information.

With the sudden increase of cases, especially narcotics cases, during the late 1960s, the federal prosecutor generated an informal policy by which the state could have a more systematic control over the plea bargaining of its cases. Specifically, deputy prosecutors are assigned to a particular court for a given length of time (approximately a year) during which they become familiar with the particular judge's sentencing and procedural policies. In this way, the prosecution can fit its case to the general temper of the judge and be in a position to give fairly accurate indications of probable sentences in a case being plea bargained. This makes plea-bargaining negotiations much more concrete and efficient for the state. Given this structure, the complaint department must distribute cases in terms of which judge is drawn on a particular case. That is, when the trial judge is drawn after the magistrate binds the defendant over for trial, the complaint department deputy simply passes the case on to the trial deputy assigned to that court.

Tactics, Procedures, and Goals of the Defense and Prosection

Plea bargaining involves several interrelated factors. First, the quality of arrest (that is, whether search-and-seizure violations occurred) affects the strength of the prosecution's case. Second, the perceived character of the defendant—that is, whether he or she is thought to be a significant member of the smuggling organization and/or has a history of past arrests—affects the negotiations. Third, the validity of the account given by the defendant is usually taken into consideration.[39] Finally, the case load of the prosecutor's office or the number of cases it must process has a bearing on the plea negotiations. Generally, plea bargaining of cases involving a cold border bust at the port of entry will be significantly different from an arrest in the field by a roving patrol or by a major undercover arrest using informants. The structure of the arrest will affect the relevancy of search-and-seizure issues, the type of person arrested (perceived character of the defendant), the probability of gaining information about other dealers (local crime patterns and police methods of apprehension), as well as the importance of accounts in generating a practical defense. Not only does the arrest affect the relative importance of these variables, but the divergent goals of the defense and prosecution significantly alter the way in which they are structured. Unlike the defense, who is concerned primarily with getting the best reduction for his or her client, the prosecution has a number of other organizational pressures affecting discretionary powers. On the one hand, the police are interested in gaining information about other dealers and pressure prosecutors to make significant reductions in order to gain this information. On the other hand, there is public pressure to curtail drug traffic through the sanctioning of drug offenders. As one experienced prosecutor stated, "We have several often conflicting pressures on us during the plea bargaining process. What we try to do is come to some sort of settlement that will be socially acceptable to all of those involved."[40]

Plea Bargaining the Cold Border Bust

Of the two types of border arrests, the port of entry or cold border bust is the most common one processed through the federal court system and is also the most mechanically structured when it is plea bargained. The arrest usually involves a mule who is very low within the drug hierarchy and/or only marginally involved in the organization. Hence, the prosecution does not take an overly punitive approach in plea bargaining because most mules are not seen as criminal types but rather as persons who are being economically exploited by drug dealers. This perception of the defendant's character is usually reinforced by the defendant's often having a large family (often five or six children), who are sometimes brought into court during sentencing. In this case, the defense counsel will often place the defendant's character as a prime focus in the plea negotiations while the prosecution will tend to underplay it but will often tend to go easy on the first offender.

Crucial to the plea negotiations is the issue of prior record. Most prosecutors and some judges are more lenient in determining an appropriate charge and sentence, respectively, if they are sure that the defendant is not a major member of the drug traffic. If there is no official information from a reliable informant or a past record indicating prior drug dealings, then the defendant's account becomes relevant in determining his position within the organization. In most cases, the defendants speak little or no English, and because the contraband was found in the possession of the defendant, the accounts are not especially elaborate. Usually a defendant will simply say he did not know that the drugs were in his car and the defense attorney will generate a probable account. One defense attorney put it this way:

> Usually, these guys speak little or no English; they are poor and have little understanding of the legal process they find themselves in. In these cases I try and find a likely way of interpreting the facts of the case so that the defendant is seen to be simply a pawn of larger dope dealers. Actually, the defendant often knows that there is "something" in the car, but is not involved in the loading of it and doesn't know much about the operation. If the facts indicate that he really did not know there was contraband, then I'll push the case. If it looks like he was just trying to make some money, I'll try and get him to turn information, otherwise it's just chancing the trial.[41]

Thus, given the structure of the arrest, the focusing on accounts as either a means of gaining an acquittal or a dismissal of charges and/or reduction of charges through painting a sorrowful picture of the defendant's plight is only moderately effective. If it is a first arrest and the facts of the case support the contention of only nominal involvement in drug traffic (for example, the defendant has no money for an attorney, the arrest report indicates no change in composure during search, or there is no information from informants on the defendant), then the prosecution is likely to give the defendant the benefit of the doubt. Most members of the court (both defense and prosecution) feel that all mules have some connection with the drug traffic, and most have engaged in smuggling prior to their present arrest. Specifically, most persons I interviewed in 1974 were aware of the use of a lie detector test by a major defense group to determine the positions of the various defendants within the drug operation. The defense attorneys in this association were forced to give up such tests because they would invariably indicate that the defendant had engaged in prior smuggling activities. Thus, most members of the court see the mule as having a connection with the drug operation, but his position is so nominal as not to warrant the full weight of the legal sanctions available on the first arrest.

Unlike the perception of the defendant's character, which may have some import in the plea-bargaining process, search and seizure is almost never an issue in a cold border bust. Procedural rules governing the search and seizure of contraband hidden in an automobile or other personal possessions are so broad as never to be an issue in court. The only point at which these issues may arise is concerning body cavity searches, and here police procedures are usually fairly sophisticated and are often supported by supervision directly by the U.S. Attorney's Office. The only other variables that may become a point of contention within the plea-bargaining situation are police needs for information. Under federal law, the U.S. attorney is required to "cooperate with local, state, and federal agencies concerning traffic in controlled substances and in suppressing the abuse of controlled substances."[42] To accomplish this end, the U.S. attorney is required to structure the plea-bargaining situation in a way that will induce any defendant to give information against codefendants, persons involved with the defendant in the smuggling operation, and/or other smugglers known to the defendant. Hence, the necessity of gaining inside information concerning criminal activities is directly and legally integrated into the plea-bargaining situation.

The low and/or marginal position of the mule, however, makes him unable to give much significant information against other members of the organization. One prosecutor explained:

Sure, if some guy wants to give me information on a whole drug operation, in short, give us the world, I'll be more than happy to dismiss all his charges. I don't care about the little guy, I want the one that is raking in all of those big profits. Although these mules usually have information to indicate possible dealers, they almost never have enough to actually turn a case. Given this, I don't see why we should make any significant reductions for this kind of information.[43]

Although mules may not be in a position to give enough information to turn a case, they are often able to provide general leads that substantiate a given investigative course being taken by federal investigators or give direction to new areas to be investigated. The federal agencies are constantly attempting to correlate and integrate information received from various low-level informants and defendants in order to determine the most productive lines of investigation. Here the information received by officials may be of some value on an accumulative basis but is not significant enough to influence the plea-bargaining process in terms of the individual cases. The use of turning information as a means of affecting the plea negotiations is more significant in cases involving relatively large dealers who have information on persons at the top of the various smuggling organizations. These persons are usually apprehended through undercover investigations in Mexico and the United States and seldom are caught at the border. Hence, there is a significant difference between the cold border bust of a mule, in which there are few variables that can be negotiated or plea bargained, and the arrest and adjudication of a major dealer that becomes the focus of intensive negotiations.

Both the prosecution and the defense understand that there is an informal and almost mechanical system through which the cold border bust can be routinely reduced in order to gain pleas of guilty. (The overall structure of this informal system is outlined in the appendix to this book and involves only the amount of contraband apprehended as the primary determiner of reductions.) The defendant's character is important in those cases in which there is a prior record, and the prosecution and defense usually are willing to increase the charge by one category for each prior arrest the defendant is known to have. For example, if the defendant has been apprehended with two kilograms of marijuana and has no known prior arrest for drug violations, he is initially charged by the complaint department with felony possession with intent to distribute and felony importation of a controlled substance. Then, within the plea negotiations he is routinely offered (and usually accepts) a reduction of the charge from two felony counts to one misdemeanor count, which reduces the possible sentence from a potential maximum of thirty years for the two felony counts (fifteen years per count) to a maximum of one year for the misdemeanor. The total fine is reduced from a potential $50,000 for the two felony counts to $1,000 for the misdemeanor. These are substantial reductions and are hard for the defense to reject given the limited area of defense caused by the lack of due process issues and the like.

A second variable affecting the negotiation of cold border busts is the perceived character of the defendant. Generally the prosecution will require that the defendant plea to the next higher category for each prior arrest the person has. The defendant with two kilograms of marijuana would have to plead to the federal possession statute (21

U.S. Code 844), which would increase the total possible penalty to one year in jail and a possible $5,000 fine. Here, the fact of a prior arrest will motivate the judge to impose a harsher, perhaps full, sentence on the defendant; thus not only is the defendant given a higher charge each time he is caught and prosecuted, but the full weight of the legal sanction is more likely to be applied.

The following is a transcript of plea negotiation concerning the arrest of a mule at the San Ysidro port of entry:

Defense Attorney: Mr. Jones? Yes, I'm representing Mr. Santos, who has been indicted for felony importation and possession of marijuana.[44]

Federal Prosecutor: Yes, come in. . . . My name is Jeff. I have the file right here.

Defense Attorney: Good, we would be willing to plead to a misdemeanor possession, if you would be willing to drop the two felony counts. And can you do anything about the sentence?

Federal Prosecutor: Okay, let's see . . . yeah, he's been found with fifteen kilos of marijuana at the border. There are no search and seizure issues in this, being a border case and all. Hmmm . . . fifteen kilos is an awful big cigarette for one's personal use!

Defense Attorney: Well, I have heard that cases of this sort are reduced on a regular basis. He has no prior and he is now in jail . . . couldn't make bond. It's been about five weeks now.

Federal Prosecutor: Okay, it seems like a straight forward case. I'll reduce it to a misdemeanor and agree to remain silent at sentencing. Your man will probably get six months and a fine . . . if he has any money.[45]

Defense Attorney: He doesn't.

Federal Prosecutor: He doesn't? Are you being retained or were you appointed? (A sly smile is noticeable.)

Defense Attorney: (He now exhibits a similar smile.) I'm retained.

Federal Prosecutor: Retained by a client that doesn't have any money . . . huuh?

Defense Attorney: (Becoming serious again.) Well, I don't know about that six months, I've read in the papers where guys are getting less time with a lot more stuff.

Federal Prosecutor: Yeah, well, the papers only give part of the story. A lot of those guys are giving information to agents and have different judges doing the sentencing. Your man happened to pull one of the harsher judges . . . he will probably get a harsher sentence with this particular charge. Although, you say he has already spent five weeks in jail, that may be enough for the judge. I can't say for sure. But I'll agree to not make any trouble and will stay quiet at sentencing.

Defense Attorney: Okay. I'll go down to the jail and do some arm twisting. I think we'll take it and I'll let you know if he objects.[46]

A number of features of this plea-bargaining situation are significant. First, the transcript exemplifies an understanding between the defense and prosecution that there is an informal and standardized system of reductions based on the amount of contraband found. Second, there is no contention concerning procedural issues, the defendant's character ("he has no prior"), the need to gain information from the defendant, or the defendant's account of the event. All of these issues are either not relevant enough even to mention or are cleared up in a brief sentence or phrase. The only formal contention is the appropriate sentence, an area of discretion beyond the control of the prosecutor. Here the defense attorney did attempt to put some pressure on the prosecutor, a common tactic in even the most open-and-shut border arrest.

Given that the reduction of charges is accomplished in a routine manner and that the defendant is primarily interested in the sentence he is likely to get, the prosecution has generated a system of negotiations concerning the relative influence the prosecution is willing to place on the judge at sentencing. Although the sentencing is legally the domain of the judge, judges routinely consult the probation department and prosecution, as well as the defense attorney and his client, to gain as much information as possible on which to base the sentence. Hence the way in which these members of the court see the defendant (his character, position in the organization, and so forth) potentially affects the outcome of sentencing. In the case under study, the prosecution was willing to remain silent and therefore reduce any negative information presented to the judge at sentencing.

The significance of such tactics in affecting the sentence is often more as a superficial ritual than a real concession by the prosecution. Although each judge does listen to all of the relevant information at sentencing, there are significant differences among judges as to the importance that is placed on this information and recommendations from the adversaries. As one senior judge stated:

Some of us take the recommendations of the prosecution seriously, but I don't. I listen to the facts presented by the probation officer in the probation report and consider the likelihood that a fine and/or jail will really stop this guy from doing it again. But I don't listen to all the rhetoric that is made by the defense and prosecution. I know what the guy should get and I give it to him.[47]

The significance of the prosecution's remaining silent varies by judge, a fact known by most experienced defense attorneys. However, irrespective of the actual importance of such a "concession," the fact that the prosecution remains silent often gives the defendant the impression that his attorney has been working actively in his favor. Thus, defense attorneys will often attempt to get the prosecution to remain silent irrespective of the known significance of such a tactic. The "arm twisting" that the defense counsel was going to do on his client in jail would be aided by the prosecution's concession to remain silent.

Finally, the transcript indicates an underlying inconsistency: defense attorney was retained by a client who was thought to be incapable of paying a fine of about $400 or $500. This incongruity brought a small amount of joviality to the situation because it points to a well-known, but not often mentioned, aspect of the adjudication of mules through the federal courts: a number of defense attorneys defend numerous federal and local drug cases and become well known among drug dealers. Although no member of the court indicates that he is on the payroll of criminal syndicates, there is widespread knowledge that these attorneys have close ties with these drug elements and are routinely hired by the organization to defend mules. One magistrate who thought the process was too close to the criminal element said:

For a while the big dealers would differentiate between those mules that had enough information on the organization to hurt them, from the naive pawns. In the case of the former they would usually pay their bail, often a four or five digit number, and the defendant would skip bail and go to Mexico. The pawn would just have to sweat it out in jail and take his chances in court. Now, they were losing a lot of money this way, so they started getting good attorneys who would charge a fraction of the bail cost and require their man to stay in jail until the adjudication process was finished. This helped them by reducing costs and the time in jail was often enough so the judge would let the mule go with time spent and a small fine. The guy that really makes out in this situation is the defense attorney who can grind through several of these cases a week, and is often down in the prosecutor's office to plea bargain before the prosecutor's office to plea bargain before the prosecutors have even received information from the border officials.[48]

As the defense attorney's reputation increases, he is called to handle more drug cases and becomes more proficient. Thus, there is an ascending cycle that makes a number of attorneys more integrated into both the plea bargaining of drug cases and drug traffickers.

The U.S. Attorney's Office almost completely controls cold border busts. The initial assignment of charges to new cases by the complaint department was based on an informal criterion that emphasized a degree of leniency relative to the total charges possible but the retaining of enough strength to induce a quick and decisive plea negotiation. There are few variables open to negotiation in such cases. The quality of the arrest, the low level of the defendant in the smuggling operation, and a well-understood system of reduction of charges leaves little to negotiate. The prosecution and defense attorney might debate the position of the defendant in the larger smuggling operation, but unless there is concrete information on other smugglers coming from the defendant, a standard reduction will be offered. In some cases, a prosecutor may offer to remain silent during sentencing, but that is a tactic more for show than an offer with actual substance.

The U.S. Attorney's Office is organizationally structured to maximize its control over most potential ambiguities in drug cases. By having all of the cases processed by the complaint department, there is an initial structural homogeneity to the offers made to defendants and their attorneys. This homogeneity reduces the possibility of a particular attorney in the office being seen as weak. Further, each trial attorney is assigned to one judge for as much as a year, which ensures the prosecutor of a close and clear understanding of the judge's courtroom procedures and sentencing style. Through this firsthand knowledge and consistent interaction, the U.S. attorney is seldom confused about the probable outcome of his or her cases. In short, the structure of the prosecution's involvement with the adjudication process, as well as the content of the plea negotiations, indicates few areas of ambiguity that are not adequately controlled by the prosecution in the cold border bust.

Plea Bargaining Cases Generated by the Roving Patrol

The plea bargaining of cases generated by the roving patrol is structured similarly to that of the cold border bust, with the exception that search-and-seizure issues are scrutinized more closely by the defense. With the necessity of either proving that the defendant was known to have crossed the border and the search was an extended border search or that the officer had full Fourth Amendment probable cause, the burden of proving the adherence to procedural stipulation falls on the prosecution. As one experienced defense attorney stated:

There isn't much to negotiate in port of entry cases, but when they nail a guy out in the boondocks, I really check that arrest report. If there is any indication that the police have overstepped procedural rules or have questionable grounds for the search or arrest, then there is something to negotiate. Usually, we can't get a full suppression of evidence on these issues, but we can get a substantial reduction of charges and perhaps some positive recommendations to the judge at sentencing. So most search and seizure issues involving the arrest and confiscation of large amounts of drugs are usually bargaining points, not a means of actually getting an acquittal or dismissal of charges.[49]

The plea bargaining of such cases is somewhat less routine and may require more complex tactics by both prosecution and defense.

On the whole, border officials tend to base the necessary probable cause on three features of the arrest situation: information existing that either the car or driver was involved in prior drug operations, the demeanor of the driver, and, in the case of large marijuana arrests, the smell of bulk marijuana. By organizing a case on one or more of these features, the police are able to control the information on the arrest report in a way that significantly buttresses the prosecution's position for plea bargaining. Again, information control within problematic situations is the key to organizational power.

When agents have prior information on the suspect, neither the police nor the prosecutor is required to divulge the specific source of such information. This gives law enforcement officials considerable leeway in constructing cases based on this type of information. As a practical matter, members of the law enforcement agencies usually collect and attempt to synthesize a large amount of fragmented information on smuggling operations. Their sources may include an informant in Mexico, an anonymous tip by phone, or information gleaned from a plea negotiation; none of these informants understand the total operation. Seldom do officers get concrete information as to the time, place, or specific persons involved in bringing contraband into this country. Hence, many times the information that is used as a basis for the arrest is simply a general hunch based on a number of fragmented tips. Such hunches or "general forms of information" have been ruled to be legal grounds for a search of an automobile or individual near the international border (*U.S.* v. *Figueroa-Espinoza*, 1972).

Second, the reference to the defendant's demeanor at the time of the search and/or arrest is a significant basis for probable cause because the officer is usually the only party in a position to determine the suspiciousness of the defendant's demeanor. The courts have ruled that nervousness per se is not grounds for probable cause for a search; however, nervousness taken in conjunction with other features of the situation can provide the basis for probable cause. Specifically, nervousness coupled with a furtive attempt to hide narcotics or marijuana from the officer's sight, indications that the car has traveled off the road (weeds in lower areas of the car) or from the direction of the border (tire tracks from the border area), and/or indication that the defendant was under the influence of drugs are all grounds when taken in toto for probable cause. Within an actual courtroom situation, it is the officer's word against that of the defendant, and the judge and/or jury is much more likely to believe the testimony of the officer. This is especially true when the officer has found and confiscated a significant amount of drugs.

Finally, in the case of bulk marijuana, officers routinely state that after stopping the suspect, who seemed suspicious, and during routine questioning, the officer smelled the "pungent odor of bulk marijuana." If the officer did in fact find bulk marijuana in a car and the car was in a place that gave the officer grounds for a stop under *Terry*, then the claim that marijuana was in evidence is an easy basis for the necessary probable cause. The routine generation of such forms of post facto rationales for probable cause would be natural, and there would be little that the defense could provide to refute such claims.

Given this and the fact that many prosecutors are aware that some of these claims made by the arresting officer may be fabricated, there is a conscious attempt on the part of some prosecutors to negotiate search-and-seizure issues in the more ambiguous cases. As a U.S. attorney stated:

Plea bargaining is an attempt to reach a conclusion to the case that is socially acceptable to all of those involved. All of the members of the court want to dispose of the case in an efficient, yet professional manner. If a defense attorney attempts to suppress evidence on every little technicality in every case, the judge will begin to wonder about his professional judgement and may informally sanction him by rejecting the majority of his motions. At the same time, the prosecutor wants to process his cases efficiently and does not want to waste time on each technicality of each case. Thus, there is pressure to negotiate those cases which involve ambiguous search and seizure issues.[50]

Here, the attorney is indicating that there is a generally understood basis as to what constitutes a legitimate search-and-seizure issue and what is an ambiguous case that should be negotiated. As each prosecutor gains experience, he or she is able to typify the kind of police accounts that will be acceptable to a particular judge. The standard accounts of smelling bulk marijuana, the suspect's demeanor, and the existence of general information are effective foundations for bringing a case to the courts.

On the whole, most members of the prosecutor's office are willing to reduce the charge one complete level (see Appendix) in cases involving an ambiguous search-and-seizure issue. However, if the officer's case is reasonably strong, they might negotiate a willingness to remain silent at sentencing in order to expedite the case but would press for the normal plea bargain and possibly a full trial if the defense was not willing to drop search and seizure issues. On the other hand, if the defense attorney feels that he must prove that he is actively pressing for his client's interests, he may make motions to suppress evidence irrespective of the probable outcome. A young attorney mentioned:

I probably won't win this motion, but the guy has paid a lot to retain me, and I feel I owe him my best. The police claim probable cause on nervousness and a furtive movement by the driver to conceal a joint and I'm going to focus on whether they could really see a furtive movement by the driver to conceal a joint and I'm going to focus on whether they could really see a furtive movement from several yards away—the distance they first spotted the car. But, like they found two hundred and fifty pounds, the judge isn't going to throw that out.[51]

Thus, there are numerous pressures surrounding the border agents, prosecutors, and defense attorneys in their apprehension and negotiation of cases between the ports of entry. Police and prosecutors have generated informal but effective ways of controlling information to buttress cases that will be plea bargained. Through the coordination of information, both within the computers and that gleaned from the field interrogation, the government is able to reduce search-and-seizure issues significantly in otherwise highly problematic situations. Although the cases generated by the roving patrol are not cold border busts, they are at least relatively strong when the inherent ambiguities are controlled in this manner.

SUMMARY

The arrest, prosecution and plea bargaining of suspected drug smugglers are structually interrelated. The effective control of information in an inherently ambiguous situation has tended to generate relatively strong cases for plea negotiations. The routinized arrest procedures at the border ports of entry create cases that can be plea bargained according to a well-understood but nevertheless informal set of charge reductions (see Appendix). The lack of significant search-and-seizure issues, the relatively low position of the mule in the smuggling operation, and the pressure on prosecutors to process cases efficiently make the plea bargaining of these cases fairly standard and routine. In the case of those apprehended by the roving patrol, however, the problem of search-and-seizure issues is more relevant, and defense attorneys are more likely to press for a significant reduction in charges in those cases in which these issues might be helpful to the defendant's case. Although cases generated by the roving patrol are much more carefully scrutinized, police and prosecutors have generated a less concrete but still relatively effective form of information control that ensures a reasonable degree of leverage within the plea bargaining situation.

4 PLEA BARGAINING LARGE NARCOTICS CASES

Thus far this book has focused primarily on the apprehension and adjudication of the small dealer-user and the mule. Now the analysis turns to the more complex, and from the perspective of the DEA, more fruitful methods of generating information on large drug dealers. Large drug dealers organize their operation so that the mule takes the most risk and receives the smallest amount of remuneration. The members of the court are not concerned with these individuals but would rather apply the full weight of the law to those who reap the most profits from the operation—those who are also the most difficult to apprehend.

THE STRUCTURE OF THE DRUG ENFORCEMENT ADMINISTRATION AND ITS USE OF INFORMANTS

"The DEA's basic emphasis in the enforcement of the law has been in stopping the flow of drugs from their foreign sources, distribution and illicit commerce at the more organized levels, and assisting state and local officials in preventing illegal drugs from reaching the community level."[1] In order to accomplish these goals the DEA has been structured as the major information-gathering and law enforcement coordinating organization within the United States. Currently there are regional offices in all of the major metropolitan areas of the United States and offices in thirty-one other countries. Generally most local law enforcement agencies tend to focus mainly on local dealer-user cases where relatively small amounts of drugs are involved. Similarly port of entry cases tend to involve small drug dealer-users of narcotics and mules importing large amounts of marijuana and seldom persons who are particularly high within the smuggling organization. Thus, the DEA acts as an information-gathering agency that collects and coordinates any information gleaned from these defendants that may yield grounds for organizing a major assault on the upper levels of drug smuggling. It is responsible for gathering, synthesizing, and disseminating information on major drug operations to the various federal, state, and local, as well as foreign, law enforcement agencies. This information is seen to provide a composite picture of the ongoing and constantly shifting structure of the various drug smuggling organizations and acts as a systematic means of attacking the traffic.

Probably one of the best modes of generating information is through pressuring a defendant to become an informant ("snitch") against his codefendants, other persons he knows within the particular drug operation, or persons known to be working within other sectors of the smuggling network. The DEA has a formal structure by which it can systematically obtain information from significant informants at the local, state, federal, or international level. Specifically, the DEA has a number of agents who work closely with specialized agencies from the narcotics units at the local levels and have information on the ebb and flow of drugs at this level. As Skolnick points out:

Local police departments, especially the vice squads, [are] proud of their relations with other law enforcement agencies. This working relationship is important for the efficient enforcement of the narcotics laws, since local, state, and federal police provide each other with complementary information.[2]

This perspective is supported by an experienced member of the DEA who had been with the Customs Department for some years prior to his present assignment:

As a rule we work as closely with the local police as necessary in making large drug arrests. They have specific kinds of information as to how much stuff is available, the time that it is likely to hit the streets, and the local dealers that have the strongest connections with the importer. We are not interested in the small time dealer, let alone the user, but these people can have information that can substantiate and round out our ideas about the larger dealers. So the local police not only can help corroborate our existing information and, hence, make our efforts more effective, but we can give them information on the larger picture that can help them in their enforcement procedures.[3]

This symbiotic relationship between local and federal agencies has become formalized with the creation of the Metropolitan Enforcement Groups (MEG), made up of several members of the DEA who are assigned to a particular metropolitan area in conjunction with a number of persons from the local narcotics squad. Through these groups information from both the federal and local levels is collated, analyzed, and disseminated.

In a similar manner, the DEA has attempted to generate strong ties with federal officials of those countries that are most heavily involved in the production and importation of drugs into the United States. The most significant traffic from the perspective of this study is the marijuana and narcotics that come from Mexico. Unlike the cooperation that is readily available from local officials within this country, the DEA's relationship with Mexican officials is somewhat more strained. Being a poor country without the strong puritanical tradition evident in the United States, there is less zeal in their attempts to control the abuse of drugs. As one official put it, "To get the Mexican police to do anything, you need either a lot of coin or a cattle prod—or both."[4] Because there is no strong moral commitment to drug control, the DEA has been forced to rely on monetary forms of motivation in its work with Mexican officials and informants. Much of the training of Mexican narcotics agents is done in the United States, and a substantial amount of money, in terms of bonuses and equipment, has gone into supporting Mexican efforts to seek out and apprehend those who produce drugs in the Mexican interior. To supplement these official channels, the DEA has a standing policy of paying Mexican informants a standard amount for a given amount of information. Although officials are reluctant to indicate the actual amount they pay for their information, they did emphasize that informants are paid on the basis of "amount of work done," not in terms of any kind of salary. Informants also are often offered various border crossing and work permits for the United States. In this way, the officials have a stable economic lever over the informant to get him to continue to provide usable information.

Whether informants are generated at the local levels within the United States or are from the drug-producing countries abroad, a number of legal issues complicate the use of their information within the courtroom. Recent rules of evidence require disclosure of all relevant evidence to both the prosecution and defense, so the problem of having to disclose the identity of a valuable informant has become a significant area of contention between prosecutors and defense attorneys. The rules of discovery require that the prosecution disclose the identity of any informant who may be able to upgrade significantly the case of the defendants. Thus, the prosecution is required to disclose the informant and make the person available for cross-examination if the defense can prove that the informant is crucial to its case. Technically, the prosecution does not have to disclose the identity of the informant if the latter is simply the vehicle of information to the police and/or prosecution. However, if the informant is actually part of the drug transaction, then the prosecution may have to produce the informer on the grounds that the informer may have been a party to the entrapment of the defendant. Entrapment or any other procedural violation is an issue that ultimately must be decided by the judge and/or jury.

To avoid this problem, the DEA has a policy of requiring that all informers remain a good distance, both geographically and temporally, from the actual drug transaction. In this way, the defense attorney will have difficulty proving that the informant was instrumental in cajoling or coercing the defendant into a transaction that he or she would have otherwise avoided. Should an informant be required to testify, the DEA will usually allow the defense to gain a dismissal of the case before revealing their informant. According to one DEA agent:

We will do everything we can to protect our informants. It is rare that they will ever have to testify. We feel that more can be gained by having them available to give us information on several transactions, than can be gotten from pressing one particular case.

At the state level, it is somewhat different. The DA will often prosecute a case and require the informant to testify in order to make his case stick. Sort of a bird in the hand is worth two in the bush philosophy. At the federal level, we want to work our way up to the big dealer and are very reluctant to lose a well placed informant on a small or mediocre case.[5]

Here the agent indicates that a large amount of information that may be gleaned from an informant is more important than a particular case that may involve entrapment issues. From a practical basis, the ultimate decision will be based on the perceived potential of the informant's information as compared to the importance of the particular case. As a rule, though, informants stay anonymous.

A number of generalizations can be made concerning the structure of the DEA law enforcement activities at the local, state, and international levels. First, the drug enforcement officials at each of the levels attempt to coordinate their information-gathering and law enforcement activities in order to maximize the efficiency of their efforts. Although there is more intranational cooperation among agencies than exists among countries, there are some undercurrents concerning jurisdiction and the granting of resources to the DEA as opposed to the other related federal agencies (such as the Bureau of Customs). Second, informants are a crucial aspect of the DEA's attempts to gain access to the more organized levels of the drug traffic. Thus, the DEA is a highly integrated feature of the plea-bargaining process at the federal level and is readily available to assist in gaining and using information from various defendants. The DEA is structured to be able to generate a coordinated program of apprehension quickly should the appropriate information be gained from a talkative defendant.

Finally, the issues of coercion and entrapment are crucial to the use of informants. Ideally the informant will be a peripheral member of the actual drug transaction or the informant will simply introduce a law enforcement officer to the drug dealers and then drop out of sight. In either case, the informer is free of court entanglements. Should the informant be in a position that would require a court appearance, however, the DEA usually will attempt to protect informants from having that particular case effectively prosecuted.

PLEA BARGAINING: THE COURTS, COERCION, AND THE CONTROL OF INFORMATION

Given the DEA's emphasis on working up the drug hierarchy, it has had to develop practical guidelines for pressuring defendants to divulge information during plea negotiations. Just as Customs was faced with the problem of integrating legal constraints into apprehension procedures, so too the DEA has had to formulate discretionary boundaries that meet Supreme Court dictates. The primary issue that has faced the DEA has been the recent Court decision concerned with illegitimate coercion during plea negotiations.

In a series of cases—*Brady* v. *United States, McCarthy* v. *United States, McMann* v. *Richardson,* and *Parker* v. *North Carolina*—the Supreme Court outlined the discretionary boundaries within which plea negotiations must take place. Specifically, the state cannot use or threaten to use physical force in order to induce information or a guilty plea. Further, under the Fifth Amendment protection against self-incrimination, any plea must be entered voluntarily. However, the state can legitimately induce a guilty plea through offers of leniency. The acceptance of these inducements is considered voluntary if the defendant has competent counsel, understands the consequences of his plea, and is not improperly coerced by the state. Justice White, speaking for the majority opinion, outlined a legitimate plea bargain:

[A] plea of guilty entered by one fully aware of the direct consequences, including the actual value of any commitments made to him by the court, prosecutor, or his own counsel, must stand unless induced by threats (or promises to discontinue improper harassment), misrepresentation (including unfulfilled or unfulfillable promises), or perhaps by promises that are by their nature improper or having no proper relationship to the prosecutor's business (e.g., bribes). *Brady vs. U.S.* (1968).[6]

Misrepresentations and improper offers can be determined by examining the legal discretionary powers of the prosecution. Under *McCarthy* v. *United States* (1969), the judge must ensure that the prosecutor's offer, and hence the final charge to which the defendant pleads, is compatible with the original charge against the defendant. That is, the prosecution must structure its offer in terms of necessarily included lesser offenses.[7] Further, any promise made by the prosecution that influences the defendant's decision to plead must be maintained in order for the plea to be accepted by the court (*Santobello* v. *New York*, 1971). Finally, the judge must obtain a verbal statement from the defendant indicating that the latter is cognizant of all the implications of his plea and has voluntarily entered the plea in light of the options open to him. Hence, the judge is responsible for determining the propriety of the prosecution's offer.

When the issues of misrepresentation and improper offers are judicially determined by an examination of the record, the problem of voluntariness may still remain problematic. The standards for assessing whether a plea is entered voluntarily have been outlined in *Parker* v. *North Carolina*, in which the Court stated that a plea is involuntary if

physical or psychological tactics employed exerted so great an influence upon the accused that it could accurately be said that his will was literally overborne or completely dominated by his interrogators, who rendered him incapable of rationally weighing the legal alternatives open to him. *Parker vs. North Carolina* (1970).[8]

To protect the defendant's constitutional rights and to ensure a voluntary plea, the Supreme Court handed down the now-classic decisions that ensure defendants of the right to an attorney (*Gideon* v. *Wainwright*), of access to that attorney at the point at which the state accuses the suspect of a crime (*Escobedo* v. *Illinois*), and of knowledge of his rights prior to entering a plea (*Miranda* v. *Arizona*). The Court attempted to ensure voluntariness (the ability to weigh rationally the legal alternatives) by ensuring competent representation to protect the defendant against illegitimate state pressure at any point in which the defendant may enter a plea. The Supreme Court, however, has not been completely clear or stringent on its definition of "competent counsel." Generally the Court has felt that "the matter, for the most part, should be left to the good sense and discretion of the trial courts" (*McMann* v. *Richardson*, 1970).[9] Unless it could be proven that the state's pressure was great enough to make the defendant "incompetent or otherwise not in control of his mental faculties," the bargain would be considered voluntary.[10]

Thus, the issue of voluntariness in plea bargaining must be analyzed in terms of these interrelated factors: the fundamental procedural rules governing the plea negotiations process, the formal and informal means of pressure at the disposal of the state, and the role of the defense attorney in protecting the defendant's right against self-incrimination. These factors will be addressed in terms of a representative transcript of a plea negotiation involving a defendant who had been apprehended for smuggling and intending to sell a large amount of cocaine. The transcript was part of a larger study done between 1973 and 1974 and conducted interviews with federal drug enforcement officials, judges, prosecutors, and defense attorneys, as well as examination of Ninth Circuit federal court records.

EXISTENTIAL-CONFLICT THEORY: THE PRACTICAL INTEGRATION OF LEGAL CONSTRAINTS AND INFORMATION CONTROL DURING PLEA NEGOTIATIONS

Plea bargaining is particularly difficult to study in depth and in a systematic way because of its ad hoc nature. Plea negotiations can take place in any number of situations: the prosecutor's or defense attorney's offices, the judge's chambers, in the corridor outside the courtroom, or over lunch in a restaurant. Not only is it difficult to locate these interactions, but court records are often incomplete. Regarding variables affecting plea negotiations—prior record, ethnicity, occupation, facts surrounding arrest, and so forth—court records do not indicate how the various factors were weighed during negotiations. Extralegal factors, such as a court's case load, public sentiment toward a particular crime, informal systems of charge reduction, and the defendant's willingness to cooperate with the state are not mentioned in court records. At best, records indicate the initial charge, some factors affecting negotiations, and the final charge accepted by the defendant. There is no indication of the exact process by which pleas are negotiated and charge reductions are structured—a process central to the issue of information control during plea negotiations.

Because of these shortcomings of official records, existential-conflict sociologists convincingly argue that one must attend to the actual social context of a situation in order to appreciate the subtle techniques used by members to further their particular interests.[11] Of specific concern here is the way members generate accounts about their access to specific resources—charge reductions and information—the value of these resources to the other members, and the authenticity of their claims to these resources. Unlike the prosecution, who has institutional access to the means of reducing charges, albeit delineated by law, the defendant's claim to having information is always subject to intensive scrutiny. Thus, it is incumbent upon the defendant to convince the prosecution that he has resources, while the prosecution has simply to indicate a willingness to negotiate.

In order to present a convincing account as well as to assess the accounts presented by others, participants in the plea-bargaining situation implicitly rely on their understanding of the background expectancies embedded in the situation. These background expectancies include the unstated knowledge members employ as a "scheme of interpretation for making [their] environment... recognizable and intelligible."[12] That is, the existential-conflict theorists argue that within a face-to-face situation, such as plea bargaining, the key form of information control involves the manipulation of the background expectancies of the situation. Information control can take a number of different forms. The control of scientific information was the central point of leverage for the moral entrepreneur. In a similar manner, the FBN consciously controlled information relating to ambiguous aspects of its organizational structure and its legal mandate to enforce the antidrug statutes. Customs went to great length to protect its hegemony over information relating to border drug traffic. Just as these individuals and organizations found information control to take on a unique form particular to their own situation, so the members of the DEA have had to develop practical forms of information control within the plea-bargaining situation. In this case, the DEA's ability to manipulate the "scheme of interpretation [with which a defendant] makes [its] environment recognizable and intelligible" is its key to organizational power. To the degree that the DEA is able to control these background expectancies, it is able to pressure the defendant to accept its conditions for a guilty plea and, more importantly, to gain information on other smugglers.

This process of manipulation is not completely cognitive, however. The knowledge of the background expectancies is important, but the way in which this knowledge is emotionally charged is of equal importance. In other words, an awareness of the legal constraints governing the negotiations, the rational assessment of the defendant's account, and a practical understanding of the law enforcement resources available are all important to the members of the DEA when negotiating with a defendant. The agent's ability to manipulate the emotional context of the situation is of equal importance. As Douglas and Johnson have stated, "Social situations are fused with, pervade, and ultimately dominate thought."[13] These existential-conflict theorists rightly emphasize the weakness of an overly "rationalized, rule governed ...[and] ordered" view of any social setting, which inevitably reflects an overly cognitive view of social reality.[14] The issue, ultimately, is not whether cognitions or emotions are the primary factor in plea negotiations but rather the way in which the DEA manipulates both the background expectancies and the defendant's emotions to glean their desired social results.

A CASE STUDY OF THE DEA'S METHODS OF MANIPULATION

Generally the most fruitful type of smuggler to pressure during plea negotiations is usually the "freelance" or middle-range smuggler. Although there is no formal structure to most transactions at this level, these individuals usually have a number of significant contacts on both sides of the border. During plea negotiations, these contacts can be set up or act as a point of entrée for officials conducting ongoing undercover work. Hence, freelance smugglers are often sources to further arrests at a relatively significant level of smuggling and a means of access to the more organized levels of international traffic.

The case examined here involved $36,000 of high-quality (80 percent pure) cocaine that the two defendants bought in Mexico and smuggled across the border to be sold to a U.S. distributor. The defendants contacted a friend and known dealer in the United States in order to sell their supply and were promised that he would introduce them to a "distributor from Chicago" (the Mafia). Unfortunately for the defendants, their friend was "working off a beef." In other words, their friend had plea bargained a reduction of his sentence on heroin charges in exchange for setting up another dealer. The defendant we studied became the next target of the DEA agents. The agents had gone to some length to convince the defendants of their membership in the Mafia. They featured the appropriate accent, dressed in expensive Italian-cut suits, and sported a new black Lincoln Continental. While negotiating the deal, the agents took the defendants to a number of expensive restaurants and indicated that money was no problem in the transaction. The defendants had had no previous contact with members of the Mafia, and so the agents were able to gain their trust by fitting the stereotyped expectations of professional criminals.

The police were able to make a procedurally legitimate arrest, therefore depriving the defense of the exclusion of any evidence. The issue of entrapment could not be raised because the defendants had made it known that they were interested in making the drug deal prior to their introduction to the police. Search-and-seizure issues were irrelevant because their discussions with police about the drug deal prior to the actual transaction and arrest easily met the criterion for probable cause. Second, the quality of the arrest enabled the prosecuting attorney to apply the highest charges that the evidence permitted (felony possession and possession with intent to sell), which gave the DEA officials a maximum of leverage in the plea-bargaining situation. Finally, the DEA official and the prosecuting attorney were interested in plea bargaining the case because since the defendant had no significant criminal record, they did not perceive her as a direct threat to society. On the side of the defense was the possibility of the defendant's divulging information on significant drug deals; this was the defense's only important point of leverage. In this particular case, the actual source of the information was the defendant's boyfriend, Butch, a dealer with wider connections than the defendant, who agreed to set up some of his connections in return for a reduction of charges against the defendant. Any delaying tactic on the part of the defense would have been counterproductive because there were no legitimate grounds for a delay, and a threat to go to trial would seal the defendant's fate with a guilty verdict.[15]

Since there was no ambiguity concerning the formal aspects of the case, the only area for negotiation concerned the informal manipulation of the plea-bargaining situation by the state and, to a lesser degree, the defense. In this vein, the prosecutor explicitly defined the prosecution's and the DEA official's interests and indicated their formal power to define the plea bargaining situation in his opening statement:

Federal Prosecutor: Okay, well, I asked the defense attorney to have you come here today. I asked him about two weeks ago. On Monday, Police William's Office[16] and also Customs expects this case to be disposed of . . . which means it's going to be pleaded. And I told the defense attorney, as he probably told you, as of this date...ahh...you know...we want something to happen. Because, since I told you before, when you were over at our office...we don't need conversation, we get a lot of that...a lot of tips and that sort of thing. We need something a little constructive. And so I wanted to know...so I could make up my mind as to what was going to happen. And at this point in time, as you are probably aware, all we have is conversations. And it doesn't make any difference to me one way or the other, because I'm not the one who's facing the charges, you are. And I understand that Butch is now supposed to be over in Mexico pricing and getting something going again.

Defense Attorney: (interjecting) Yeah, Butch called me this morning.

Federal Prosecutor: Again, it's conversation; we haven't seen anything yet. We get phone calls and informed, but the defense attorney says that he understands that there is something different in that...well, why don't you tell me what is happening, before I go ahead.

The prosecutor's opening statement defined the background expectancies of the plea-bargaining situation in terms of several parameters. First, the prosecution and the various law enforcement agencies had an organizational consensus to offer to negotiate the case. Second, the prosecutor indicated the importance of the defendant giving constructive indications that a setup was going to happen, while presenting a personal indifference to the plight of the defendant. This presentation acted to establish the prosecutor and the DEA official as having a united front (which was not always the case)[17] and made it incumbent on the defendant to generate an account concerning her intentions to cooperate. For an account to be accepted by the evaluating members (DEA agent and prosecutor) it must incorporate readily understandable and sufficiently congruent information that fits the background expectancies of these members. In this endeavor, the defense attorney acted as both a mediating and a supporting agent as the defendant presented her account:

Defendant: We're trying a whole lot of other things...because we can't get anything in Mexicali before Monday. It's there that a lot of things are happening. Instead, I have this friend in Laguna Beach that is working on something. He and Butch have gotten together...it could have happened this morning, except that Butch was in Mexicali. I was sitting up all night. They were sitting up by their phone wondering why, you know, we aren't there.

DEA Agent: What's suppose to happen in Laguna?

Defendant: They have at least five pounds of cocaine...and access to people that are working on it.

Federal Prosecutor: Do you know the sources?

Defendant: Yeah, his first name is Ken. I already have his name and phone number.

Defense Attorney: Let me relate what Butch said. He called me about 9:30 this morning. He said he was in Mexicali...said he had met with his connection, Frank, at 7:00 this morning and will return to our office this afternoon and tell us what was going to happen. I told him we wanted to negotiate for four or five kilos of cocaine. They'll do it by boat trip and they'll do it from Ensenada. And that's all I can say at this point. And I'll let you both know at 3:30 what's happening. He mentioned something else about Laguna, but that's all I know about it.

Federal Prosecutor: When was the last time you heard from Butch?

Defense Attorney: It was this morning.

Federal Prosecutor: When prior to that?

Defense Attorney: About five days prior to that, he called Frank and then me.

Federal Prosecutor: Okay, then, that makes good sense. But he did call Frank?

Defense Attorney: Yeah, he did. But I was out of town, I was in Ventura.

Federal Prosecutor: Well, that's good, because that's what he told me through the defendant, that he had tried to reach you but you weren't in and then he finally did talk to Frank. And I was beginning to wonder just how much you were putting everybody on.

Defendant: (interjecting over ongoing conversation) We are frantic. It's not as easy as you would like to think it is. We are doing everything, you know.

DEA Agent: I'll be honest. I had had my doubts on how panicked Butch really was. But maybe, well, as I say, I have my doubts about it.

Federal Prosecutor: Yes, our problem is that we get this all of the time. We get people who say, "Yeah, I can turn the world for you" but you wait and wait forever. You never see anything.

The defendant was concerned with presenting herself as a frightened and cooperative suspect with a number of connections that were being exploited on both sides of the border. However, her account was somewhat unorganized and lacked specificity as to names, dates, and times because she was both frightened and a member of the drug subculture, which is not overly concerned with such details. The defense attorney volunteered this information because he understood the DEA's need for specific information that would facilitate the activation and coordination of police agencies in these two areas. The defense attorney was acting on his understanding of the background expectancies latent in this type of plea negotiation and had become an agent-mediator between the state and his client. However, this role was not necessarily detrimental to his client's interests. Rather, the presentation of such information corroborated his client's contentions that she was doing everything possible and increased her credibility and thus, ultimately, her bargaining position. Hence, the role of the defense attorney functioned within the background expectancies of the state, but while accomplishing this it could also become a source of support and precision for the defendant's account.

The prosecutor was not completely convinced that the account accurately reflected the activities of the boyfriend, Butch. Given the fact that the actual setup was being generated by Butch, misinformation might have been generated by Butch (the source) and/or by the defendant or defense attorney (the intermediaries). The prosecutor had no direct access to Butch (for the latter's protection), but he attempted to verify the validity of the defense attorney's account in terms of information about Frank, the Mexicali connection. The prosecutor had already been told by the defendant that Butch had contacted a dealer in Mexicali (Frank) and that the message had been given to the defense attorney. By pressing the defense attorney for verification of this, the prosecutor was able to determine to his satisfaction that the defense attorney's information coincided with his background expectancies based on what the defendant had told him previously. Hence, because of the adversary nature of the situation, the presentation of accounts by the defense was always subjected to evaluative scrutiny based on the state's background expectancies.

Now that the situation was clearly defined and the defendant's account validated, the next stage of the negotiations involved the prosecutor's pressuring of the defendant to generate a setup within a specific time period:

Defendant: Well, can't I have a few more days?
Federal Prosecutor: Well, now this is what I would propose. See, as far as I am concerned it won't make much difference one way or the other. But on

Monday you come in and plead and between that time and the sentencing—which is usually four weeks—you can do anything you want. You can work as much as you want during those four weeks .And, of course, anything that happens, you know, during that time would definitely be brought to the court's attention.

Defendant: Is it more difficult after that time, after the plea?

Federal Prosecutor: No ... ahh ... I don't think it makes any difference. Really what I would do is after you plead, you would only have, how many counts is it, two?

Defendant: Yes.

Defense Attorney: Yes.

Federal Prosecutor: Well, we would drop it to one count and any further help you could be will be noted to the court. It would be noted that the defendant has cooperated with the agents and here is what she has done: boom, boom, boom.

Defense Attorney: What you're not being told is that, when you plead to a felony, you can end up with five years in prison.

DEA Agent: Yeah.

Defense Attorney: Once you plead there is no way of working off your beef. There is no way of getting it reduced. Or dismissed. That's how it works out. You are pleading as charged.

Defendant: Why don't you postpone this thing Monday until Wednesday?

Federal Prosecutor: No, the agents have heard that "it will be next week", "it will be next week", "it will be a couple more days", "couple more days". And that's all we've heard, see? Not only that, but you're behind an awful lot of cocaine, you know. And that, you know, for us to even consider reducing it to a misdemeanor, I mean, you'd have to be crazy ... I mean that's a lot of stuff.

Defendant: Well, give me some idea.

Federal Prosecutor: Well, what I'm saying ... ahh ... I mean, I'm not going to ...

Defendant: You mean I should do everything I can ...?

Federal Prosecutor: Well, yeah, that's right. Everything you can. I'm not going to say that if you make five cases or if you make three cases or something like that. Because that's sort of an arbitrary thing.

The essence of this form of manipulation involved keeping the defendant off balance by trading on her emotional insecurities about her fate. The most obvious means of accomplishing this was with references to the severity of the defendant's situation in statements like, "You're behind an awful lot of cocaine." However, the interaction between the prosecutor and the defense attorney, the latter ostensibly there to protect the defendant's rights, was a much subtler point of pressure. The prosecutor outlined an offer in which she could plead to one count the following Monday, and should she generate a setup prior to sentencing (approximately four weeks away) she might gain some leniency during sentencing. Both the DEA agent and the prosecutor had a background expectancy that the defense attorney would then clarify the ramifications of the prosecutor's offer. By explaining the background of the situation (an assured sentence of up to five years in prison if a setup was not made over the weekend), the defense attorney not only presented himself as working in his client's favor but indicated there was nothing he could do within the parameters set by the prosecutor, and this prospect made a significant impact on the defendant.[18]

Of crucial importance is whether such tactics rendered the defendant incapable of weighing the legal alternatives open to her and hence comprised illegitimate forms of gaining information and/or a plea. Although the defendant's feelings were inextricably intertwined with her cognitive appraisal of her situation, there was no indication that she was incapable of weighing her options. In fact, her defense attorney clarified these options for her and acted as a cognitive counterbalance to the increasing emotional pressure placed on her by the prosecutor. Although her attorney did not reduce the emotional pressure on her, he did function to maintain her cognitive awareness of the legal alternatives open to her.

Another form of emotional pressure involved the prosecution's control over the system of charge reductions. After the case had been settled, the defense attorney indicated that both he and the prosecutor shared a background expectancy that each setup would yield a one-count reduction in the charges against the defendant.[19] But

it is in the clients' interests to keep these things quiet. If they know that a particular set up will get "X" reduction, they aim for the minimal amount and often don't bring in the goods. It is better for all concerned to leave it open-ended and get them to bring in as much as possible. Besides, who's to say the prosecution won't back down on a verbal deal, then I'd really look stupid.[20]

A final form of psychological pressure to keep the defendant off balance is illustrated in the next section of the transcript and involves the alternation between the initial hard line presented by the prosecutor and the more conciliatory line developed later by the DEA agent. Immediately after the exchange concerning the prosecutor's offer, the DEA agent interjected:

DEA Agent: I hate to be hardhearted about it, but that's just the facts of life. We have people in here who get caught with a lot less than you did . . . and pick up the felony charge. You just happened to involve yourself with a tremendous amount of narcotics. And that's just the facts of life. And I would encourage you, you know, to help act to get this thing going. Because Monday is the day.

Defendant: But it's so hard, I can only do what I can do. I'm supporting Butch. I've given him everything. He has twenty-four hours to put into this. I don't know if he is totally insane or doesn't understand the importance of this. I don't know, I haven't been around him in a long time. He seems to be very dingy . . . I try to sit him down and say, "What is happening?" and he says, "Don't worry, I've got this and this and this going." So finally I went and found this other one I have, working in Laguna Beach. And he doesn't want to be involved, he wants to give it to Butch so he won't be involved personally. So I have to wait for Butch because he was supposed to have a meeting with him at nine o'clock this morning . . . but I get a call from Butch saying, "Oh, I'm down in Mexicali." And I said, "What are you doing?" You know, I get totally frustrated, but then too, I don't want to blow it, because he will hang up and I'll never see him again. But I have so little control over him.

DEA Agent: Well, see, you've got a problem. But there is nothing that we can do about the problem. And furthermore, relating this case to other cases, we have people with similar problems . . . like your defense attorney had a guy who got caught with a ton of weed . . . a ton of weed. And the guy is sitting in jail now and the agents don't want to let him out. So the question is, how can he be cooperative when he can't get out of jail?

Defendant: (interjecting) You mean he can't get bail?

Federal Prosecutor: Now don't you worry about that.

DEA Agent: (simultaneously) Now don't you worry about that.

Federal Prosecutor: But anyway, what I'm saying is that there are people that have similar problems and they're all picking up the felonies. I mean, if you can't make it, you can't make it. Really, you are doing us a favor and in return for the favor we'll do you a favor. And if you can't do us any favors, then, that's it.

Defendant: I feel that something is there . . . because I have talked to . . .

DEA Agent: Let me put in here for a second. As far as the agents go, I'm willing to go twenty-four hours around the clock, six days. I don't care how many days it takes to get the thing done. I want to get it off the street. I'm not that particularly interested in your particular case or anybody else's case. We're willing to do it, but we have to have something to do it with. And if you can get the stuff together, even tonight, we'll rip it off. We'll rip it tomorrow or Sunday, but we've got to have something to work with.

Defendant: Fine, all right, okay.

Federal Prosecutor: That's cool. Now understand what you've got to do?

Defendant: Yeah, I've understood for months... ha, ha.

Federal Prosecutor: Well, you understand that you've got to deliver, and if you deliver, we can get you time.

Defendant: Okay.

Federal Prosecutor: And if you don't deliver, we'll send you to the judge. It's getting to the point where they're almost all the same because of the pressure on them from Washington. Okay?

Like the prosecutor, the DEA agent maintained pressure with references to the tremendous amount of narcotics involved in this case and that "there is nothing we can do about the problem." However, he presented a more flexible front and attempted to cajole the defendant by indicating that he was willing to make this a special case if the defendant acted "to get this thing going." Ironically, the DEA official almost undermined his own presentation by relating the defendant's case to that of the guy caught with "a ton of weed." The agent was implying that they have control over who gets out on bail, when in fact the judge has final discretion in these matters. The defendant, having become somewhat familiar with the criminal justice system, queried the agent: "You mean he can't get bail?"[21] This prompted the agent and prosecutor to close ranks simultaneously and terminate that line of discussion; "Now don't you worry about that." Here the defendant used background expectancies to disrupt the ritual equilibrium of the agent and prosecutor's team presentation—an equilibrium that both sides reinstituted immediately after the disruption. In the final part of this section, the defendant continued to present herself as working on a setup, the prosecutor took the hard line, and the agent reiterated his willingness to work with the defendant. The plea-bargaining session was then formally terminated.

During this interaction the defense attorney did nothing to undermine the state's pressure against the defendant. Rather, the legal alternatives had been clearly delineated previously, and the state officials were concerned with creating a level of emotional tension that would adequately motivate the defendant to generate the setups. The prosecutor ended the discussion by determining whether the defendant actually understood her position at that point and the options open to her; she indicated that she did. Again, there is evidence that her emotional state, although intense, had not undermined her ability to understand her legal alternatives.

Throughout the negotiations, the defense attorney acted as an agent-mediator to clarify the defendant's account and to make explicit the implications in the offers presented by the state. This functioned to support the defendant's understanding of her legal alternatives within the highly emotional context of plea negotiations. However, the defense attorney shifted his tactics and put significant emotional pressure on the defendant as they walked from the courthouse:

Defense Attorney: Last time we talked to them they were all ready to go, and you were going to get credit for it, and the prosecutor said, "Yeah, I'll catch hell, but okay, go ahead"... and then, at that moment they thought it was coming down that night and they stood by...
Defendant: I know...
Defense Attorney: And there was nothing. I'm surprised that they are still even willing to see you. The only reason they are still willing is because they know that Butch has a hell of a lot. You've got to deliver. Also, that stuff that they were telling you about sentencing... big stinking deal, pleading to a felony. You'll have a felony on your record, you'll be an ex-felon for the rest of your life. Every time you try to get a job and they ask you if you have ever been convicted. Yes, they can bust you down to five years, but if they bust you down to a misdemeanor then it's a maximum of one year. And all of the good things that go with a misdemeanor as opposed to a felony. Or there is the possibility that you can work it off. They are still making noises about you working the whole thing off.
Defendant: Okay, if I do this, I had better get off.
Defense Attorney: Call me up. Call me on this telephone and I will be there. Remember, it's all very, very unpleasant. Remember the people you dealt with in jail?
Defendant: Yeah...
Defense Attorney: Well...
Defendant: See, you do not understand, I am in shock... I have been in shock since I walked out of jail the other day.

Defense Attorney: Do you see what's happening?

Defendant: I don't feel good, but I have been doing everything I could do.

Defense Attorney: Get Butch to work, that's the first thing you can do. You've got to admit that when you think back to it, every time you make contact with these guys it's always promises. We're going to do this, we're going to do that, you know, that's what it always comes down to. Always walking in there making promises, and I am really amazed that they are willing to put up with it. I got this guy who's got more than a ton of weed who is screaming to cooperate and they're telling him they don't want him to cooperate.

Defendant: I know.

Defense Attorney: Here he is *screaming*, and in your case here they are standing by and willing to work twenty-four hours a day. That's incredible of them, you know. And that's because they figure that there is going to be something there, but if there isn't anything there . . .

Defendant: I know it may seem that I'm not working, but . . .

Defense Attorney: (interrupts) Yes, it really does.

Defendant: Well, I can only do my best. If I blow it he will leave for a year or so and I can't do anything.

Defense Attorney: Well, if anything happens, call me.

Defendant: Okay.

Here the defense attorney reiterated the main points presented by the state: their willingness to negotiate this case in spite of her apparent lack of cooperation, the fact that other defendants were not being offered the same opportunities, and that the only alternative to setting up a case was jail and a criminal record. Here, the member of court who was supposed to be most supportive of the defendant's interests threw his weight in support of the state's definition of the situation—by this time a very salient definition for the defendant.

CONCLUSIONS

The Supreme Court has stated that a plea is legitimate only when the defendant is able to weigh rationally the legal alternatives available and determine the option most suited to his or her interests. Given that the state has a number of ways to pressure a defendant, the free and rational entering of a plea is often problematic. This analysis has focused on the forms of pressure the DEA places on a defendant's pleading in drug cases and specifically has emphasized the interplay between the cognitive (rational) and emotional aspects of this situation. It was found that there is an intricate interplay between the members of the plea-bargaining situation in which substantial pressure is applied to the defendant, but attempts are made to ensure the defendant's complete awareness of the available legal alternatives.

There are essentially three stages in these negotiations: the members' initial presentations and definitions of the situation, the manipulation of the defendant to accept the state's guidelines for action, and the acquiescence of the defendant to the state's requests. In the opening section, the state and defendant presented information (accounts) indicating a negotiated settlement was possible; however, the defendant's account concerning her willingness to cooperate needed further validation. The defense attorney supplied this corroboration by focusing on the background expectancies of the state officials and clarified the defendant's activities prior to the negotiations. The next stage involved the pressuring of the defendant by constant references to the amounts of drugs involved, remaining vague on the specific structure of charge reductions, and alternating between a hard and soft line during the negotiations. Here again the defense attorney acted as an agent-mediator and clarified the legal ramifications of the prosecution's first offer, a clarification that motivated the defendant to cooperate with the state. Finally, the defendant overtly agreed to cooperate within a specified time period and explicitly indicated she understood the full range of options open to her. During this period, the defense attorney acted as a clarifying agent for both the state and defendant and did not overtly increase or reduce the psychological pressure on her. However, outside of the courtroom, her attorney did increase the pressure on her and reiterated the basic contention of the state.

This analysis indicates that within the plea-bargaining situation feelings are fused with and pervade thought, but the members of this situation are careful that these feelings do not completely dominate thought and hence create a basis for an appeal. The interplay between thought and emotions is complex and often problematic. However, in the case of plea negotiations, competent members of the courts have found ways to use feelings to motivate defendants to fit the goals of the state but have organized this process in ways that meet the legal requirements of the Constitution.

CONCLUSIONS

This analysis has attempted to present a new and comprehensive approach to understanding the drug issue: the existential-conflict perspective. Like any other theoretical structure, this perspective can be traced back to the works of a number of major sociological contributors (Marx, Michels, Weber, and more recently, Gusfield, Douglas, and Collins). The central theoretical ground for this tradition lies in the acceptance of the inherently problematic nature of social reality, the way in which groups and individuals generate strategies to manipulate the ambiguous social state for their own purposes, and the information feedback loops that develop when this manipulation process is successful. Within each aspect of the drug issue (the drug experience itself, the laws created for its control, and the practical drug enforcement procedures) this basic paradigm was evident.

The problematic nature of the drug experience itself was vividly reflected in the descriptions of major literary figures, as well as by members of the medical profession. Although there was considerable conflict over the proper role of drug use by the turn of this century, the negative definition of drug use predominated. The successful domination of the antidrug definition was due to the infusion of larger structural tensions (specifically class and racial hostilities) into the antidrug stereotype. Local, state, and national political figures generated the image of the dope fiend, an image that meshed easily with negative middle-class stereotypes of racial minorities. Both the dope fiend and the Chinese, black, and Mexican minorities were depicted as lazy, pleasure seeking, and potentially violent. What was of concern to the middle class was their fear of the encroachment of both drugs and minorities into the sanctuary of middle-class respectability. Just as minorities were moving into the industrial cities to find work at the turn of the century, so the middle class envisioned a steady, if not completely visible, expansion of drug use throughout society. Specifically, the antidrug mythology suggested that the unsuspecting member of the middle class could initially become habituated to a weak intoxicant, such as tobacco or alcohol. This could then create an uncontrolled desire for more pleasure and eventually lead to addiction to drugs such as opium and cocaine. Central to this simple, salient, and stable fear was the middle-class terror of the idea of losing one's will and self-control. Whether that control was undermined by drugs or the encroachment of minorities into the previously pure domain of the middle class, the deep emotional response was the same.

The larger structural tensions due to increased minority visibility, which were aggravated by economic downturns just prior to the passage of antidrug legislation, had to be integrated into the cognitive image of the dope fiend. Although the interface between these unrelated, but pervasive, social fears and this stereotype was somewhat problematic, the moral entrepreneur was able to integrate them successfully. Central to this process of integration was the strategy of working within the ecological and cultural conditions that bring individuals together for an emotional encounter, coordinating the resources for an emotional display, and controlling the accumulated techniques for emotional manipulation. Collins terms the totality of the strategies and tactics used in the process as the *means of emotional production*. The successful moral entrepreneur was the individual who could effectively use this process to infuse his desired stereotype with the intense emotions generated from these pervasive social tensions.

Although their respective geographical and cultural environments differed, both Hamilton Wright and Harry Anslinger were able to infuse the dope fiend stereotype with the deep emotional fears of minority subcultural domination of the larger class structure (Wright with Chinese and blacks and Anslinger with Mexicans). Wright worked on the international level with conferences concerning the problem of opium in the Far East and opium and cocaine within this country. Anslinger's efforts focused on the passage of the Marijuana Tax Act and worked within the geographical boundaries of this country. Regardless of their respective boundaries, both successfully coordinated the resources for an emotional display ("facts concerning the drug problem") and with that display manipulated public emotions for the passage of the desired legislation. The result was a negative feedback loop that differentiated drug users from the larger public and placed the FBN as the central source for "factual" information processing, as well as the primary agency for social control. Hence, the collective work of Wright and Anslinger successfully placed a new federal organization at the apex of the drug information processing system.

This pivotal position was further enhanced through a number of other organizational strategies designed to increase information control. Specifically, the FBN generated its organizational policies based on Supreme Court decisions that were favorable to a punitive legal approach to the drug problem. The ambiguity surrounding a number of conflicting court rulings gave the bureau a problematic setting in which to expand its organizational jurisdiction. The bureau also strengthened its political ties with key congressional committees. During the early 1950s, the bureau was able to fine tune its information control system with a series of emotional displays both within the mass media and before these congressional committees. In this particular case, the emotional tensions involved fears of inner-city blacks, the Mafia, and international communism. Although the objects of the fears differed, the legal results were the same: increased antidrug legislation.

However, by the late 1960s, the cultural climate had changed and the FBN came under its first major attack. Because of the civil rights movement, economic affluence, and a large number of liberal youths, the established negative feedback loop between the dominant white society and the minority drug user came under successful questioning. The bifurcation between whites and minorities, which allowed the FBN to control the dope fiend stereotype, began to break down due to the new image of minorities based on equal rights and, ultimately, black and Chicano power. White youth became concerned about minority rights and eventually integrated with minority activity—drug use. However, the social meaning of this activity had undergone considerable change during this decade. Rather than the dope fiend stereotype generated by the early moral entrepreneurs, new prophets in favor of drug use advocated "tuning in, turning on, and dropping out." A new cultural setting created by a war in

Southeast Asia, the civil rights movement, and a generation hooked on the mass media set the stage for a new set of moral entrepreneurs. These moral entrepreneurs, like their predecessors, knew how to control the resources for an emotional display (new "facts" about the drug experience) and coordinate the techniques for emotional manipulation (mass media). With this massive increase in the positive feedback loop for drug use, the law enforcement agencies had to respond in a new way.

Predictably, this response came with a desire by federal agencies to control the flow of information. The FBN was initially reorganized into the Bureau of Narcotics and Dangerous Drugs (1967) and again changed to the Drug Enforcement Administration (1973). With each of these transformations, there was an attempt to increase the effectiveness of information control over the drug situation. This attempt to centralize information into one federal agency met stiff resistance from other federal bureaus, especially the U.S. Customs, which already had an information processing system. Although their conflicts over computer systems, legal jurisdictions, and drug enforcement strategies have not completely abated, each agency has developed somewhat effective strategies within their particular domains.

Paramount to drug enforcement strategy is the creation of a feedback loop between smugglers and the federal law enforcement officials. Ideally state officials attempt to control the information flow so that the suspect can be identified, evidence for a conviction can be generated, and information on other smugglers can be made available. As was seen with the creation of these antidrug laws, law enforcement practices rely heavily on the manipulation of problematic situations and the intense emotions inherent in them.

In fulfilling primary responsibility of interdiction at the international border, Customs has generated a comprehensive and practical system of apprehension that integrates legal guidelines with the practical manipulation of the suspect's emotions to generate a solid court case—the cold border bust. Through their use of computerized information, informal typifications, and subtle psychological pressures, Customs officials are able to control the information flow within the border-crossing situation. Because of their broad discretionary power and accurate understanding of nervous behavior, they are able to filter out suspected smugglers from the millions of people who pass through the ports of entry each year. Customs agents structure the information feedback loop so that the psychological pressure on the suspect becomes manifest in clues that lead to his or her arrest and eventual conviction.

If the structuring of information is central to the apprehension of smugglers, it is no less crucial to the plea negotiations that follow. Here again, the federal agents—in this case, U.S. attorneys—structure a problematic situation to enhance their position of power. Ideally, an accused smuggler should be tried by his peers, but for efficiency prosecutors are willing to negotiate a guilty plea in exchange for a reduction of charges. Given that 90 percent of the cases are adjudicated in this manner, prosecutors have given considerable attention to structuring this situation in an efficient manner. They have reduced areas of ambiguity within their adjudication procedures in a number of ways, all of which involve the control of the information flow. Specifically, the U.S. Attorney's Office makes standardized initial plea offers within their complaint department so that cases are assured some uniformity. Further, each attorney is required to work for approximately one year with a particular judge to gain knowledge about the informal courtroom and sentencing style of that judge. These two strategies ensure that an initial uniformity exists among these cases but that when unique circumstances arise, the prosecutor will have the most information on the informal courtroom factors that might affect the case. Finally, in the case of the cold border bust, the plea negotiations are standardized to a degree that enables both the prosecution and the defense to negotiate the case in a relatively routine manner. Cases generated between the ports of entry or involving body cavity searches at the ports of entry may involve some negotiations over possible procedural violations in the field, but usually these negotiations are not extensive. The feedback loop between suspect and Customs agent is usually simple, salient, and stable enough to ensure a strong case for the prosecution.

If cases generated by Customs at the ports of entry are handled in a routine manner, the DEA cases are usually more complex. Because the DEA bases its organizational strategy on gleaning information from plea negotiations, its officials have developed complex tactics to keep the defendant emotionally motivated to turn new cases.

Through the judicious control of background expectancies, the prosecutors and DEA agents are able to gain information from local, state, and federal plea-bargaining situations enabling them to set up and, they hope, to arrest the most significant members of larger drug rings. Some of these tactics include keeping the rules of the negotiations problematic, indicating a lack of interest in the defendant's plight, and alternating between a hard and conciliatory line of questioning. Irrespective of the particular tactics involved, their strategy, like the other members of the drug scene, is to control information in ambiguous situations to maximize their capacity for forming an information feedback system desirable to them. Because of the nature of social reality, such systems will ultimately be created, only to break down eventually and require reorganization. However, as long as individuals desire experiences out of the ordinary and feel that drugs are the most effective means for gaining these experiences, there will be state organizations attempting to control these individuals.

APPENDIX
Standardized System of Charge Reduction Informally Generated by the U.S. Attorney's Office

A. **Misdemeanor Charge**
   1. *A few marijuana cigarettes to one kilogram (2.2 pounds).*

      Cases falling within these limits are routinely given an informal form of diversion. Under federal law (Title 21, U.S.C. 844b), any person who has not been convicted of a narcotics violation and is found guilty or pleads guilty to this section—possession of a controlled substance—with consent of the court, may be deferred for a probationary period of up to one year. During this period, the defendant must meet certain probationary conditions (for example, not be arrested for a narcotics violation, give up Fourth Amendment rights, and not be in the company of any known dealers or users), upon the successful completion of which his case will be dismissed and all records of the proceedings expunged, except for one nonpublic record of the divergence kept for the sole purpose of ensuring that a defendant will be given only one divergence.

      Federal prosecutors indicate a willingness to divert hard narcotics involving up to approximately three grams of heroin or cocaine.

   2. *One to five kilograms of marijuana*

      Cases involving these amounts of contraband are routinely plea bargained to a state health and safety code violation (11357) that involves misdemeanor possession with a maximum of six months in jail (county jail) and a $500 fine. The federal courts are able to incorporate any state law into their criminal justice system, under Title 18 U.S.C. 13, thus giving a large body of statutes from which to structure a system of plea bargaining reductions. This particular statute was chosen because of its relatively low fine when compared to the federal possession statute of a misdemeanor with one year in jail and a $5,000 fine.

In terms of hard narcotics, prosecutors are willing to reduce charges to the health and safety code violation (11357) in cases involving up to one half ounce of cocaine or heroin.

3.   *Five to ten, and possibly fifteen, kilograms of marijuana.*

Cases involving these amounts of marijuana are offered a reduction from the initial full possible charge given by the complaint department to the federal statute (Title 21 U.S.C. 844) of misdemeanor possession. This carries a maximum of one year and $5,000. Prosecutors indicate that they will routinely reduce cases involving up to ten kilograms to this possession charge, but between ten and fifteen kilograms exists a gray area. Most U.S. attorneys will try to get a felony conviction or plea on over ten kilograms, but will reduce if there are mitigating circumstances, such as a heavy case load that week or procedural issues.

In the case of heroin or cocaine, defendants with one-half to one full ounce will also be given this reduction.

B.   Felony Charge

1.   *Above fifteen kilograms of marijuana.*

Cases involving large amounts of marijuana are usually required to plea to a felony charge of "possession with intent to distribute" (Title 21 U.S.C. 846). In most of the standard cases involving a large amount being brought across the border by a mule, the initial charge will include possession with intent to distribute and the related charge of illegal importation of a controlled substance (Title 21 U.S.C. 952); and if there is evidence of more than one person being involved, the appropriate conspiracy charges are added (Title 21 U.S.C. 960). In such cases, the plea negotiations will usually focus on the dismissal of the latter charges for a plea to the basic possession with intent to distribute, and the dismissal of three felony counts for the plea to one felony count—yielding a reduction of the maximum sentence from sixty years in prison and $100,000 fine for the full four counts to fifteen years in prison and $25,000 on the one count of possession with the intent to distribute.

In the case of hard narcotics, the same offer is made for any amount above one ounce.

Generally, the prosecution will make these reductions for all cases in which the defendant is not known to have a prior record, with a number of qualifying situations. First, if the defendant is known to be a dealer but was caught with only a small amount, prosecutors will push for the full charge—plead as charged or go to trial. Second, if the defendant is known to have a prior record, there will be an effort to get a plea to the next highest category in the schedule. For example, if he has one prior arrest and is caught with nine kilograms of marijuana, he will be offered a plea to the one count of felony possession with intent to distribute rather than the misdemeanor possession. Generally, each prior offense will knock the appropriate charge up at least one more notch. In some cases, prosecutors will want to become extremely hard bargainers and require pleas to felony on all second offenses. It is much less routine, and much more bargaining is involved, in cases involving several prior offenses.

NOTES

INTRODUCTION

1. Jack D. Douglas, *Drug Crisis Intervention, A Report to the National Commission on Marijuana and Drug Abuse* (Washington: Government Printing Office, 1974), p. 34.

2. Howard Becker, "Marijuana: A Sociological Overview," in *The Marijuana Papers*, ed. David Solomon (New York: Mentor Books, 1966), pp. 76-78.

3. Jack D. Douglas, *The American Social Order* (New York: Free Press, 1971), p. 142.

4. Albert Hess, "Deviance Theory and the History of Opiates," *International Journal of the Addictions*, vol. 6, no. 1 (1971):585-98.

5. Carol Warren and John Johnson, "A Critique of Labelling Theory from the Phenomenological Perspective," in *Theoretical Perspectives on Deviance*, ed. Robert Scott and Jack Douglas (New York: Basic Books, 1972), p. 90.

6. The most significant empirical studies by these existential-conflict theorists include: Jack Douglas, *The Social Meaning of Suicide* (Princeton, N.J.: Princeton University Press, 1968); Aaron Cicourel, *The Social Organization of Juvenile Justice* (New York: John Wiley & Sons, 1968); Carol Warren, *Identity and the Gay Community* (New York: Wiley-Interscience, 1974); John Johnson, *Doing Field Research* (New York: Free Press, 1975); and Jack Douglas and Paul Rasmussen, *Nude Beaches* (Beverly Hills, Calif.: Sage Publications, 1977).

7. Randall Collins, *Conflict Sociology* (New York: Academic Press, 1975), p. 7.

8. Ibid., p. 11.

9. Randall Collins, "A Comparative Approach to Political Sociology," in *State and Society: A Reader in Comparative Political Sociology*, ed. Reinhard Bendix (Boston: Little, Brown, 1968), p. 51.

10. Collins, *Conflict Sociology*, p. 153.

11. Jack Douglas, *Existential Sociology* (New York: Cambridge University Press, 1977), p. 15.

12. Jack Douglas, "An Existential View of Man in Society: The Dominance of Feeling in Human Life" (unpublished manuscript, 1976), in ibid., p. 8.

13. Joseph Gusfield, *Symbolic Crusade* (Urbana, Ill.: University of Illinois Press, 1972), p. 180.

14. Ibid., p. 4.

15. Ibid., pp. 179-80.

16. Ibid., p. 4.

17. Ibid., pp. 5-6.

18. Ibid., p. 5.

CHAPTER 1

1. Thomas De Quincey, "Confessions of an English Opium Eater," in *The Forbidden Game*, ed. Brian Inglis (New York: Charles Scribner's Sons, 1975), p. 111.

2. Thomas De Quincey, "Confessions of an English Opium Eater," in *The Drug Experience*, ed. David Ebin (New York: Orion Press, 1961), pp. 120-21.

3. William Blair, "An Opium Eater in America," in Ebin, *Drug Experience*, p. 42.

4. Ibid.

5. Ibid.

6. Ibid., p. 134.

7. Ibid.

8. Ibid., p. 133.

9. Ibid., p. 135.

10. One of the many tragic ironies of history was that one of the first to become addicted to morphine through the use of the hypodermic needle was the wife of its inventor, Dr. Alexander Wood of Edinburgh, Scotland. The invention was thought to avoid the problem of "opium appetite" due to the oral ingestion of the drug. Although the hypodermic needle has been a major benefactor for modern medicine, Mrs. Wood proved the error of the "opium appetite" perspective. See Charles Terry and Mildred Pellens, *The Opium Problem* (Montclair, N.J.: Patterson Smith, 1928), pp. 65-67.

11. T. D. Crothers, "Morphinism and Narcomania from Other Drugs," in Terry and Pellens, *Opium Problem*, p. 69.

12. W. G. Smith, "On Opium Embracing Its History, Chemical Analysis and Use and Abuse as a Medicine," in Terry and Pellens, *Opium Problem*, p. 61.

13. E. G. Eberle and F. T. Gordon, "Report of Committee on the Acquirement of Drug Habits," in Terry and Pellens, *Opium Problem*, p. 106.

14. Jack Douglas, *Drug Crisis Intervention, A Report to the National Commission on Marijuana and Drug Abuse* (Washington: Government Printing Office, 1972), p. 42.

15. Sigmund Freud, "Cocaine Papers," in *Cocaine Papers*, ed. Robert Byck (New York: Stonehill, 1974), p. 9.

16. Ernest Jones, *The Life and Work of Sigmund Freud* (New York: Basic Books, 1961), 1:63.

17. Ibid., p. 54.

18. Richard Ashley, *Cocaine: Its History, Uses, and Effects* (New York: St. Martin's Press, 1975), p. 49.

19. Quotation from Sir Arthur Conan Doyle, "Scandal in Bohemia" in ibid., p. 38.

20. Ibid.

21. Quotation from Sir Arthur Conan Doyle, "The Sign of the Four" in Ashley, *Cocaine*, p. 39.

22. Charles Baudelaire, "Les paradis artificiels," in Ebin, *Drug Experience*, p. 20.

23. Ibid.

24. Ibid.

25. Bayard Taylor, "The Land of the Saracen or Picture of Palestine, Asia Minor, Sicily, and Spain," in Ebin, *Drug Experience*, p. 61.

26. Ibid., p. 49.

27. Ibid., p. 50.

28. Quoted in Solomon Snyder, *Uses of Marijuana* (New York: Oxford University Press, 1971), p. 11.

29. Quoted in ibid., p. 15.

30. C. Towns, "The Injury of Tobacco," *Century*, (March 1912):22.

31. Quoted in Stanford Lyman, *The Asian in the West* (Las Vegas, Nev.: Western Studies Center, Desert Research Institute, 1970), p. 18.

32. Frank Soule, John Gihon, and James Nisbet, *The Annals of San Francisco* (Palo Alto, Calif.: Lewis Osborne, 1966), pp. 378-79.

33. H. H. Kane, *Opium Smoking in America and China* (New York: G. P. Putnam, 1882), p. 4.

34. Richard Blum and Associates, *Society and Drugs* (San Francisco: Jossey-Bass, 1970), p. 53.

35. Terry and Pellens, *Opium Problem*, p. 808.

36. C. Vann Woodward, *The Strange Career of Jim Crow* (New York: Oxford University Press, 1957), pp. 82-86.

37. Ibid., pp. 67-68.

38. Lawrence Kolb, "Drug Addiction in Its Relation to Crime," *Journal of Mental Hygiene*, vol. 9, no. 1 (January 1925):88.

39. E. G. Eberle and F. T. Gordon, "Report of Committee on the Acquirement of Drug Habits," in Terry and Pellens, *Opium Problem*, p. 107.

40. Quoted in John Helmer, *Drugs and Minority Oppression* (New York: Seabury Press, 1975), p. 47.

41. Quoted in ibid., pp. 47-48.

42. R. S. Copeland, "The Narcotic Drug Evil and the New York City Health Department," in Terry and Pellens, *Opium Problem*, p. 851.

43. Richard Bonnie and Charles Whitebread, *The Marijuana Conviction* (Charlottesville: University Press of Virginia, 1974), p. 33.

44. Helmer, *Drugs and Minority Oppression*, p. 61.

45. Quoted in ibid., p. 59.

46. Quoted in Bonnie and Whitebread, *Marijuana Conviction*, p. 34.

47. My analysis focuses on Durkheim's work because he made the most significant classical statement on functionalism and the most explicit use of the law as a reflection of predominant social values. Parsons, Merton, and some lesser theoretical figures have contributed to the area of the sociology of law, but their most significant theoretical contribution can be traced back to the original work by Durkheim. By focusing on the most salient aspects of his theory, a general appreciation and critique of the functionalist contribution to this area can be made. See Emile Durkheim, *The Division of Labor in Society* (New York: Free Press, 1933), p. 79.

48. Ibid., p. 79.

49. Ibid., p. 63.

50. Joseph Gusfield, *Symbolic Crusade* (Urbana: University of Illinois Press, 1972), p. 114.

51. Jack Douglas, *The American Social Order* (New York: Free Press, 1971), p. 139.

52. I have used Becker almost exclusively to describe the moral entrepreneur or labelling theory and Lindesmith in a later section dealing with labelling theory and the Harrison Act. I have concentrated on these two authors because I believe they were the first and the clearest of those espousing this theoretical viewpoint. This, of course, is not meant to detract from the others in this area. Many have contributed to the understanding of drugs and the law, but both Becker and Lindesmith remain at the apex of this area of scholarship. See Howard S. Becker, *The Outsiders: Studies in the Sociology of Deviance* (New York: Free Press, 1963), p. 147, and Alfred Lindesmith, *The Addict and the Law* (Bloomington: Indiana University Press, 1965).

53. Randall Collins, "The Empirical Validity of the Conflict Tradition" in *Contemporary Sociological Theory*, ed. Allan Wells (Santa Monica, Calif.: Goodyear Publishing Co., 1978), p. 185.

54. Randall Collins, "A Comparative Approach to Political Sociology," in *State and Society: A Reader in Comparative Political Sociology*, ed. Reinhard Bendix (Boston: Little, Brown, 1968), p. 51.

55. Carol Warren and John Johnson, "A Phenomenological Critique of Labelling Theory," in *Theoretical Perspectives of Deviance*, ed. Robert A. Scott and Jack D. Douglas (New York: Basic Books, 1972), p. 73.

56. Collins, "Empirical Validity," p. 185.

57. David Musto, *The American Disease* (New Haven: Yale University Press, 1973), p. 33.

58. Ibid.

59. Ibid.

60. Gusfield, *Symbolic Crusade*, p. 170.

61. Collins, "Empirical Validity," p. 185.

62. Quotation from Hamilton Wright's *Report on the International Opium Commission and on the Opium Problem as Seen Within the United States and Its Possessions* in Helmer, *Drugs and Minority Oppression*, p. 47.

63. Ibid., p. 63.

64. "Second International Opium Conference" in Terry and Pellens, *Opium Problem*, p. 641.

65. Ibid., p. 753.

66. Ibid., p. 754.

67. Ibid., p. 755.

CHAPTER 2

1. Randall Collins, *Conflict Sociology* (New York: Academic Press, 1975), pp. 315-16.

2. Jack Douglas and John Johnson, *Existential Sociology* (New York: Cambridge University Press, 1977), p. 50.

3. "United States v. C. T. Doremeus, T. D. 2809" and "W. S. Webb and Jacob Goldman v. United States, T. D. 2809," in Charles Terry and Mildred Pellens, *The Opium Problem* (Montclair, N.J.: Patterson Smith, 1928), p. 759.

4. "Pro-mimeograph No. 217, October 19, 1921" in Terry and Pellens, *Opium Problem*, p. 757.

5. "United States v. C. T. Doremeus, T. D. 2809" and "W. S. Webb and Jacob Goldman v. United States, T. D. 2809," p. 759.

6. Alfred Lindesmith, "Federal Law and Drug Addiction," *Social Problems*, vol. 7, no. 1 (Summer 1959): 49.

Lindesmith's work on the Harrison Act and the Supreme Court decisions that followed is considered to be the most comprehensive and articulate statement to date. Most other scholars refer to this original statement in their work. See Edwin Schur, *Crimes Without Victims* (Englewood Cliffs, N.J.: Prentice-Hall, 1965), and Troy Duster, *The Legislation of Morality* (New York: Free Press, 1970).

7. *Lindner v. United States*, 268 U.S. 189 (1925).

8. Ibid.

9. Collins, *Conflict Sociology*, p. 216.

10. Alfred Lindesmith, *The Addict and the Law* (Bloomington: Indiana University Press, 1965), p. 143.

11. Michael Crozier, *The Bureaucratic Phenomenon* (Chicago: University of Chicago Press, 1964), p. 196.

12. Howard Becker, "Marijuana: A Sociological Overview," in *The Marijuana Papers*, ed. David Solomon, (New York: Mentor Books, 1966), p. 97.

13. James C. Munch, "Marijuana and Crime," *United Nations Bulletin on Narcotics*, vol. 18, no. 2 (1951):23.

14. The major sociological study that has attempted to determine the relationship between drug use and cultural violence is Herbert Blumer's study of Oakland, California, ghetto youth and the use of marijuana. Blumer found that there were at least two ghetto subcultures: the "rowdy gangs ... which may be characterized as aggressive, boisterous, wild, and undisciplined. They are disposed towards fighting, seizing on any drug, but generally prefer marijuana." In contradistinction to this group is the "cool culture which emphasizes being unruffled in critical stituations, keeping one's head, showing calm courage, and controlling one's behavior. The members of the cool culture are further subdivided into pot heads, mellow dudes, and players. All use marijuana and none are aggressive physically." See Herbert Blumer et al., *The World of Youthful Drugs* (Berkeley: University of California Press, 1964), p. 88.

15. Roger Smith, "U.S. Marijuana Legislation," *Journal of Psychedelic Research*, vol. 1, no. 3 (1968):108.

16. U.S. Treasury Department, Bureau of Narcotics, *Traffic in Opium and Other Drugs for the Year Ending December 31, 1937* (Washington: Government Printing Office, 1938), p. 39.

17. Collins, *Conflict Sociology*, p. 316.

18. John F. Galliher and Allynn Walker, "The Politics of Systematic Research Error: The Case of the Federal Bureau of Narcotics and a Moral Entrepreneur," *Crime and Social Justice* (Fall-Winter 1978–1979):29-33.

19. John Helmer, *Drugs and Minority Oppression* (New York: Seabury Press, 1975), pp. 60-61.

20. Ibid., p. 61.

21. Paul S. Taylor, "Crime and the Foreign Born: The Problem of the Mexican," in ibid., p. 212.

22. Helmer, *Drugs and Minority Oppression*, p. 74.

23. Ibid., p. 103.

24. Testimony of Harry Anslinger before the United Nations Commission on Narcotic Drugs, 10th Sess. April-May 1955, reprinted in U.S. Congress, House, Ways and Means Committee, Subcommittee on Illegal Drug traffic, *Traffic in and Control of Narcotics, Barbiturates, and Amphetamines*, Hearing, 84th Cong., 1st Sess., October-December, 1955 (Washington: Government Printing Office, 1955), p. 200-203.

25. Helmer, *Drugs and Minority Oppression*, p. 74.

26. Ibid., p. 117.

27. Howard Becker, *The Outsiders* (New York: Free Press, 1963), pp. 85-86.

28. Quotation taken from *Minneapolis Tribune*, February 11, 1938, cited by Richard Bonnie and Charles Whitebread, *The Marijuana Conviction* (Charlottesville: University of Virginia Press, 1974), p. 185.

29. Collins, *Conflict Sociology*, p. 314.

30. Ibid.

31. Richard Ashley, *Cocaine: Its History, Uses and Effects* (New York: St. Martins Press, 1975), p. 95.

32. James Carey, *The College Drug Scene* (Englewood Cliffs, N.J.: Prentice-Hall, 1968), p. 38.

33. Aldous Huxley, *Doors to Perception* (London: Chatto & Windus, 1968), p. 20.

34. Ibid, p. 52.

35. Alan Watts, *Joyous Cosmology* (New York: Pantheon Books, 1962), p. 70.

36. Ibid., p. xiii.

37. Howard Becker and Irving Horowitz, *Culture and Civility in San Francisco* (New Brunswick, N.J.: Transaction Books, 1972). This gives the most complete description of the social order within San Francisco at the time referred to.

38. Carey, *College Drug Scene*, p. 12.

39. Ibid., p. 28.

40. Quoted in Fred Leavitt, *Drugs and Behavior* (Philadelphia: W. B. Saunders Co., 1974), p. 52.

41. Henry Giordano, Commissioner of Narcotics, report to U.S. Congress, House, Committee on Public Health and Welfare, Subcommittee on Drug Abuse, *Increased Controls over Hallucinogens and Other Dangerous Drugs*, Hearing, 90th Cong., 2d Sess., March 19, 1968 (Washington: Government Printing Office, 1968), p. 106.

42. Carey, *College Drug Scene*, p. 39.

43. Giordano, *Increased Controls*, p. 107.

44. Ibid., p. 108.

45. Ibid., p. 109.

46. Ibid., p. 108.

47. Carey, *College Drug Scene*, pp. 172-206.

48. Jack D. Douglas, *Drug Crisis Intervention* (Washington: Government Printing Office, 1974), pp. 74-75.

49. Albert Goldman, *Grass Roots: Marijuana in America Today* (New York: Harper & Row, 1979), p. 94.

50. Hank Messick, *Of Grass and Snow: The Secret Criminal Elite* (Englewood Cliffs, N.J.: Prentice-Hall, 1979), p. 50.

51. Collins, *Conflict Sociology*, p. 318.

52. U.S. Comptroller General, report to U.S. Congress, House and Senate, *Illegal Entry at United States-Mexico Border: Multiagency Efforts Have Not Been Effective in Stemming the Flow of Drugs and People* (Washington: Government Printing Office, 1977), p. 19.

53. U.S. Congress, House, Committee on Narcotics Abuse and Control, *Oversight Hearings on Narcotics Abuse and Current Federal and International Narcotics Control Efforts*, Hearing, 94th Cong., 2d Sess., September 21-30, 1976 (Washington: Government Printing Office, 1977), p. 445.

54. The local and state law enforcement communications system, termed NLETS (National Law Enforcement Telecommunications System), coordinates all relevant information among local jurisdictions and helps coordinate law enforcement tactics at the local level. The FBI's National Crime Information Center (NCIC) makes federal cases and information available to local and state law enforcement agencies. Given the national distribution system through which drugs are disseminated, Customs's information concerning border interdiction would be greatly facilitated by being integrated with the data banks of these two information systems.

55. Committee on Narcotics Abuse and Control, *Oversight Hearings,* p. 444.

56. Ibid., p. 455.

57. Ibid.

58. Comptroller General, *Illegal Entry*, p. 30.

59. Ibid., p. 29.
60. Committee on Narcotics Abuse and Control, *Oversight Hearings*, p. 319.
61. Ibid., p. 318.
62. Comptroller General, *Illegal Entry*, p. 24.
63. Ibid., p. 47.
64. Ibid., p. 48.
65. Ibid., p. 49.
66. Ibid., p. 48.
67. Ibid., p. 50.
68. Collins, *Conflict Sociology*, p. 328.
69. Ibid.

CHAPTER 3

1. U.S., Congress, House, Select Committee on Narcotics Abuse and Control, *Interdiction of Drug Trafficking in Louisiana*, Hearing, 96th Cong., 1st Sess., November 19, 20, 1979 (Washington: Government Printing Office, 1980), p. 47.
2. Drug Enforcement Administration, *Drug Enforcement*, Winter 1975-1976, pp. 37-38.
3. Quotation is taken from an interview with a border official in 1974. All transcript quotes are from my research in the border area around San Diego, California, between June 1973 and July 1974. The names of officials are confidential; only the individual's role (border official, judge, prosecutor, and so forth) is identified.
4. The terms *border officials, federal law enforcement officers*, and *federal officials* include not only Customs officials and federal narcotics officers but also Immigration and Naturalization officials insofar as they are involved in apprehending drug smugglers while enforcing alien laws.
5. A senior member of the DEA quoted this figure during interviews. Although there is no way that the government can know exactly the percentage of smugglers caught, this member of the administration indicated that the percentage was very low—approximately 5 percent.
6. Quotation taken from an interview with a federal official in 1974.
7. Only those ports of entry between Mexico and California were studied; officials indicated that apprehension techniques were essentially the same along the entire border.
8. Information received from interview with border official in 1974.
9. Boyd v. United States, 116 U.S. 616 (1886).
10. Carroll v. United States, 267 U.S. 134 (1924).

11. These three cases—*Terry*, *Mapp*, and *Chimel*—constitute the basic procedural guidelines governing police search-and-seizure powers over citizens within the United States.

Terry v. Ohio, 392 U.S. 1 (1968), governs initial police-citizen contact. It ruled that "in justifying a particular intrusion, the police officer must be able to point to *specific and articulable* facts which, taken together with rational inference from those facts reasonably warrant that intrusion"(italics added). Hence, an officer must glean a specific and articulable set of facts from a situation to legitimate stopping a person and patting down the exterior of that person in search of weapons. This scope of police powers is equivalent to a "founded suspicion" governing the border officials' powers over persons crossing the Mexican-American border.

Mapp v. Ohio, 367 U.S. 643 (1961), established the general exclusionary rule that requires both state and federal police to adhere to Fourth Amendment requirements of probable cause to legitimate the search and seizure of private property. Should this criterion be violated, the defense can have the illegally seized evidence excluded from the trial.

Chimel v. California, 89 S. Ct. Repts. 2034 (1969), outlines police search-and-seizure powers during a lawful arrest. Whereas *Terry* is concerned with a simple police stop and *Mapp* indicates the necessity of probable cause to search a person when the officer does not have enough evidence for an arrest, *Chimel* outlines the limits of a search in cases where there is enough evidence for an arrest. Specifically, "a warrant must be obtained in all cases in which there is ample time," and an officer may conduct a limited search without a warrant only in "areas within the immediate control of those being arrested." Hence, the Court is limiting the power of police to extend a search arbitrarily into any area that cannot be directly and immediately tied to the defendant.

12. Landau v. United States, 82 Fed. 2nd (1936).

13. Alexander v. United States, 362 Fed. 2nd (1966).

14. Thomas v. United States, 372 Fed. 2nd (1967).

15. Jack Douglas, *Understanding Everyday Life* (New York: Aldine Press, 1970), p. 9.

16. Henderson v. United States, 390 Fed. 2nd (1967).

17. Case taken from federal court docket and arrest report. The examples used in this section were derived from three different sources: information extracted from arrest reports and/or court records, examples given by members of the court during interviews, and data derived from information received while attending actual trials and pretrial hearings. I selected the cases use in this chapter on the basis of their being the most closely related to the analytical point being made and were the richest in detail that would further clarify the analysis.

18. Data interpolated from an interview with an experienced defense attorney.

19. Unlike the local police, the federal drug enforcement agencies do not publish a written report indicating the exact number of persons arrested for narcotics violations. However, a count of two separate two-week periods of the cases presented in the federal court docket provides a fairly accurate representation of the number of cases adjudicated by the courts. This is exemplified by the following breakdown of drug arrests during two two-week periods in 1973:

	January 1-16, 1973	*June 18-July 5, 1973*
Total cases of all kinds	439	417
Total drug cases	252	213
Marijuana cases	130	126
Heroin cases	48	51
Cocaine cases	17	13
Pills casses	16	14
Other controlled substances	41	27

These figures are not exact because of an unknown number of cases in which arrests were made but no charges were brought by the U.S. attorney at the initial stages, and/or the court informally diverted the case and the record was sealed upon fulfillment of the diversion. This example shows that marijuana cases make up the bulk of the drug cases at the border. Heroin is next, and pills and cocaine are last. The apprehension of large amounts of hard narcotics is usually done by the DEA through undercover and informant operations, while the port of entry cases are primarily marijuana cases.

20. Paraphrased from notes taken during a federal preliminary hearing.

21. This physiological indicator of the age of track marks is not an absolute and infallible means of determining how recently a person has used the needle. Some persons who do not heal at a normal rate may have oozing or red openings for some time after the injection. However, from a legal perspective, the members of the court assume a normal rate of healing unless the defense can prove otherwise.

22. Quotation taken from an interview with a senior border official in 1974.

23. Title 8 U.S. Code 1357a.

24. Title 8 C.F.R. 287.1.

25. Quotation taken from an interview with a border official in 1973.

26. Quotation taken from an interview with a U.S. attorney in 1974.

27. Paraphrased from notes taken during a federal preliminary hearing.
28. Quotation taken from an interview with a federal magistrate in 1974.
29. Quotation taken from an interview with a deputy U.S. attorney in 1974.
30. Title 21 U.S. Code 844.
31. Title 21 U.S. Code 841a.
32. Title 21 U.S. Code 846.
33. The amount of contraband seized is the primary indicator that the defendant was probably interested in selling it. If there is more than one kilo or less than a kilo and it is broken down into lids (bags of five or six ounces), this is usually enough to motivate the prosecution to make the charge a felony.
34. Usually such information is informally received through informants or from law enforcement officials who have been watching a particular person for some time prior to the arrest.
35. Title 21 U.S. Code 846.
36. Title 21 U.S. Code 952.
37. Quotation taken from an interview with a senior federal prosecutor in 1974.
38. This statement is the result of a general impression I developed after interviewing a wide range of law enforcement officers and members of the state and federal courts. No statistical data support this claim, but almost everyone I interviewed indicated that the federal officials were more flexible in their plea-bargaining policies than were the state prosecutors.
39. Stanford Lyman and Marvin Scott, *The Sociology of the Absurd* (New York: Appleton-Century-Crofts, 1970), p. 112, describe an account as a "linguistic device employed whenever an action is subjected to evaluative inquiry." Obviously accounts become a significant part of the plea-bargaining situation, and the quality of the account is a significant factor in determining the quality of a prosecution or defense case.
40. Quotation taken from an interview with an experienced federal prosecutor in 1973.
41. Quotation taken from an interview with an experienced defense attorney in 1974.
42. Title 21 U.S. Code 873.
43. Quotation taken from an interview with a federal prosecutor in 1974.
44. In this transcript, the names are fictitious, but the dialogue is an actual plea-bargain negotiation between a federal prosecutor and a defense attorney.
45. A follow-up on this case indicated that the bargain was accepted by the defendant and the case was disposed of as agreed upon in this transcript. The

defendant was sentenced to one year in jail, six months suspended, and a $1,000 fine.

46. Transcript of plea negotiations between defense attorney and federal prosecutor.

47. Quotation taken from an interview with a senior judge in 1973.

48. Quotation taken from an interview with a federal magistrate in 1973.

49. Quotation taken from an interview with a defense attorney in 1974.

50. Quotation taken from an interview with a defense attorney in 1974.

51. Quotation taken from an interview with a defense attorney just prior to a preliminary hearing in 1974.

CHAPTER 4

1. *Drug Enforcement Administration Fact Sheet* (Washington: U.S. Government Printing Office, 1973), p. 4.

Much of this chapter is reprinted from my article, "Prosecution's Power, Procedural Rights, and Pleading Guilty: The Problems of Coercion in Plea Bargaining Drug Cases," *Social Problems,* vol. 26, no. 4 (April 1979): 452–66. All copyrights are the property of the Society for the Study of Social Problems, and this part of the article is made available here through the permission of the society.

2. Jerome Skolnick, *Justice Without Trial* (New York: John Wiley & Sons, 1966), p. 143.

3. Quotation taken from an interview with a DEA investigator in 1973.

4. Quotation taken from an interview with a DEA official with twenty-five years of experience in the southern California area in 1974.

5. Quotation taken from an interview with a DEA official in 1974.

6. Brady v. United States, 379 U.S. 752 (1968).

7. Necessarily included lesser offenses are offenses that must be committed in order for a suspect to have committed the crime for which he or she is charged. For example, petty theft is necessarily included in burglary, and possession of a controlled substance is necessarily included in attempting to sell controlled substances. Situationally included lesser offenses are those in which the suspect engaged in lesser crimes while engaging in the offense for which he or she is being held. For example, battery is not necessarily included in burglary, but it may be a lesser charge in some cases. For a detailed description of how these categories affect the routine plea bargaining of cases at the state level, see D. Sudnow, "Normal Crimes," In *Deviance: The Interactionist Perspective,* ed. E. Rubington and S. Weinberg, (New York: Macmillan, 1973).

8. Parker v. North Carolina, 396 U.S. 759 (1970).

9. McMann v. Richardson, 397 U.S. 759 (1970).

10. Brady v. United States, 397 U.S. 752 (1968).

11. The research for this chapter took place in a federal circuit court contiguous with the Mexican-American border and was conducted between January 1973 and August 1974. During this period there were intensive in-depth interviews conducted with all of the judges and magistrates of the court, all of the federal prosecutors who handled drug cases on a regular basis within the district, several DEA agents, and about twenty-five well-known and respected defense attorneys who dealt with drug cases. The particular DEA officials and defense attorneys were chosen through referrals made by judges, prosecutors, and other defense attorneys.

During this period, I obtained several transcripts of plea-bargaining negotiations, but these were usually of a very routine nature involving mules or low-level dealer-users. Understandably the members of the court were reluctant to give an outsider access to the more sensitive negotiations that yield significant amounts of information concerning other dealers. I am indebted to a defendant who was able to tape her plea negotiations and make that tape available to me. The findings of that tape were then used as a basis for interviews, which allowed me both to clarify the nature of the background expectancies and to verify the universality of the tactics manifest in the tape.

This transcript involves a case where arrest procedures used by the DEA precluded search-and-seizure issues being available to the defense. The primary issue in the transcript involves the extralegal negotiation of information in exchange for a charge reduction and, more importantly, the tactics used by the state to gain the defendant's cooperation during negotiations. Subsequent interviews with other members of the court indicate that the transcript is representative of most other negotiations involving drugs.

12. Aaron Cicourel, *The Social Organization of Juvenile Justice* (New York: John Wiley & Sons, 1968), p. 15.

13. Jack D. Douglas and John M. Johnson, *Existential Sociology* (New York: Cambridge University Press, 1977), p. 38.

14. Ibid., p. 56.

15. In cases involving third-party (citizen) witnesses and legitimate grounds to contest the procedures used in the arrest, it is reasonable for the defense to engage in pretrial motions or delaying tactics; witnesses' memories begin to fade, witnesses become harder to locate, and much of the evidence may be excluded on procedural grounds. Further, by threatening to go to trial, the defense can tie up the court's calendar and use court resources in a lengthy trial. However, this is a poor tactic in cases where a guilty verdict is

likely because courts are known to be quite harsh on those who refuse to plea bargain, use court court resources, and then have the case resolved in favor of the state.

16. This case was generated by the DEA but with the help of local police ("Police William's Office"). Although the DEA organized and set up the arrest, it was done within the jurisdiction of Officer William's department, and therefore his consent was necessary for the case to be pleaded.

17. A study of the heroin traffic between Mexico and Chicago revealed "far too many petty jealousies, suspicions, and ill feelings among law enforcement groups" (*Mexican Heroin*, Illinois Legislative Investigating Commission, printed by The State of Illinois, 1976, p. 52). For psychological and financial reasons almost every agency involved in a drug arrest wants the recognition for the work, a basic source of these intergroup ill feelings.

18. When I interviewed the defendant after the plea-bargaining session, she said, "Man, when they both [prosecutor and defense attorney] said I could get five years, man, I got scared... I knew I had to do something."

19. That is, each arrest in which the setup involves approximately the same amount of drugs that the defendant is being arrested with would yield a reduction of charges by one count. Being charged with two counts (one count of possession, one of possession with intent to sell), no arrest would get her a reduction of one count (felony possession) in exchange for an expedient plea of guilty. One good arrest and a guilty plea would reduce the charge to misdemeanor possession. Two good arrests would get her case dismissed. As the case progressed, she ultimately got the latter deal.

20. Quotation from taped interview with defense attorney on April 17, 1974.

21. The defendant knew that most smugglers who do not get bail are Mexican mules who have little useful information for the DEA and would flee to Mexico if they were temporarily released. The DEA agent was implying that he was willing to give her case special consideration; however, her response indicates that she knows hers is not a special case, and therefore the DEA agent and the prosecutor simultaneously close that line of interaction.

BIBLIOGRAPHY

BOOKS

Ashley, Richard. *Cocaine: Its History, Uses and Effects.* New York: St. Martin's Press, 1975.

Becker, Howard. *The Outsiders: Studies in the Sociology of Deviance.* New York: Free Press, 1963.

Becker, Howard, and Irving Horowitz. *Culture and Civility in San Francisco.* New Brunswick, N.J.: Transaction Books, 1972.

Bendix, Reinhard. *State and Society: A Reader in Comparative Political Sociology.* Boston: Little, Brown and Co., 1968.

Blum, Richard, and Associates. *Society and Drugs.* San Francisco: Jossey-Bass, 1970.

Blumer, Herbert. *The World of Youthful Drugs.* Berkeley: University of California Press, 1964.

Bonnie, Richard, and Charles Whitebread. *The Marijuana Conviction.* Charlottesville: University of Virginia Press, 1974.

Byck, Robert, ed. *Cocaine Papers.* New York: Stonehill, 1974.

Carey, James. *The College Drug Scene.* Englewood Cliffs, N.J.: Prentice-Hall, 1968.

Cicourel, Aaron. *The Social Organization of Juvenile Justice.* New York: John Wiley & Sons, 1968.

Collins, Randall. *Conflict Sociology.* New York: Academic Press, 1975.

Crozier, Michael. *The Bureaucratic Phenomenon.* Chicago: University of Chicago Press, 1964.

Douglas, Jack D. *The American Social Order.* New York: Free Press, 1971.

——— . *Drug Crisis Intervention.* Washington: Government Printing Office, 1974.

——— . *The Social Meaning of Suicide.* Princeton, N.J.: Princeton University Press, 1968.

——— . *Understanding Everyday Life.* New York: Aldine Press, 1970.

Douglas, Jack D., and John Johnson. *Existential Sociology.* New York: Cambridge University Press, 1977.

Douglas, Jack D., and Paul Rasmussen. *Nude Beaches.* Beverly Hills, Calif.: Sage Publications, 1977.

Douglas, Jack D., and Robert A. Scott. *Theoretical Perspectives on Deviance.* New York: Basic Books, 1972.

Durkheim, Emile. *The Division of Labor in Society.* New York: Free Press, 1933.

Ebin, David, ed. *The Drug Experience.* New York: Orion Press, 1961.

Goldman, Albert. *Grass Roots: Marijuana in America Today.* New York: Harper & Row, 1979.

Gusfield, Joseph. *Symbolic Crusade.* Urbana: University of Illinois Press, 1972.

Helmer, John. *Drugs and Minority Oppression.* New York: Seabury Press, 1975.

Huxley, Aldous. *Doors to Perception.* London: Chatto & Windus, 1968.

Inglis, Brian. *The Forbidden Game.* New York: Charles Scribner's Sons, 1975.

Johnson, John. *Doing Field Research.* New York: Free Press, 1975.

Jones, Ernest. *The Life and Work of Sigmund Freud.* New York: Basic Books, 1961.

Kane, H. H. *Opium Smoking in America and China.* New York: G. P. Putnam, 1882.

Leavitt, Fred. *Drugs and Behavior.* Philadelphia: W. B. Saunders Co., 1974.

Lindesmith, Alfred. *The Addict and the Law.* Bloomington: Indiana University Press, 1965.

Lyman, Stanford. *The Asian in the West.* Las Vegas, Nev.: Western Studies Center, Desert Research Institute, 1970.

Lyman, Stanford and Marvin Scott. *The Sociology of the Absurd.* New York: Appleton-Century-Crofts, 1970.

Messick, Hank. *Of Grass and Snow: The Secret Criminal Elite.* Englewood Cliffs, N.J.: Prentice-Hall, 1979.

Musto, David. *The American Disease.* New Haven: Yale University Press, 1973.

Rubington, E., and S. Weinberg, eds. *Deviance: The Interactionist Perspective.* New York: Macmillan, 1973.

Schur, Edwin. *Crimes Without Problems.* Englewood Cliffs, N.J.: Prentice-Hall, 1970.

Skolnick, Jerome. *Justice Without Trial.* New York: John Wiley & Sons, 1966.

Snyder, Solomon. *Uses of Marijuana.* New York: Oxford University Press, 1971.

Solomon, David, ed. *The Marijuana Papers.* New York: Mentor Books, 1966.

Soule, Frank, John Gihon, and James Nisbet. *The Annals of San Francisco.* Palo Alto, Calif.: Lewis Osborne, 1966.

Terry, Charles, and Mildred Pellens. *The Opium Problem.* Montclair, N.J.: Patterson Smith, 1928.

Vann Woodward, C. *The Strange Career of Jim Crow.* New York: Oxford University Press, 1957.

Warren, Carol. *Identity and the Gay Community.* New York: Wiley-Interscience, 1974.

Watts, Alan. *Joyous Cosmology.* New York: Pantheon Books, 1962.

Wells, Allan, ed. *Contemporary Sociological Theory.* Santa Monica, Calif.: Goodyear Publishing Co., 1978.

PERIODICALS

Galliher, John F., and Allynn Walker. "The Politics of Systematic Research Error: The Case of the Federal Bureau of Narcotics and a Moral Entrepreneur." *Crime and Social Justice* (Fall-Winter 1978-1979): 29-33.

Hess, Albert. "Deviance Theory and the History of Opiates." *International Journal of the Addictions,* vol. 6, no. 1 (1971):585-89.

Kolb, Lawrence. "Drug Addiction in Its Relation to Crime." *Journal of Mental Hygiene,* vol. 9, no. 1 (January 1925):88.

Lindesmith, Alfred. "Federal Law and Drug Addiction." *Social Problems* (Summer 1959):59.

Munch, James C. "Marijuana and Crime." *United Nations Bulletin,* vol. 18, no. 2 (1951):23.

Smith, Roger. "U.S. Marijuana Legislation." *Journal of Psychedelic Research, vol. 1, no. 3 (1951):108.*

Towns, C. "The Injury of Tobacco." Century (March 1912):22.

GOVERNMENT PUBLICATIONS

Drug Enforcement Administration. *Drug Enforcement Administration Fact Sheet.* Washington: Government Printing Office, 1973.

————. *Drug Enforcement.* Washington: Government Printing Office, 1976.

U.S. Congress. House. Committee on Narcotics Abuse and Control. *Oversight Hearings on Narcotics Abuse and Current Federal and International Narcotics Control Efforts.* Hearing, 94th Cong., 2d Sess., September 21-30, 1976. Washington: Government Printing Office, 1977.

————. House. Select Committee on Narcotics Abuse and Control. *Interdiction of Drug Trafficking in Louisiana.* Hearing, 96th Cong.,

1st Sess., November 19-20, 1979. Washington: Government Printing Office, 1980.

———. House. House Ways and Means Committee, Subcommittee on Illegal Drug Traffic. *Traffic in and Control of Narcotics, Barbiturates, and Amphetamines.* Hearing, 89th Cong., 1st Sess., October-December, 1955. Washington: Government Printing Office, 1955.

———. House. Committee on Public Health and Welfare, Subcommittee on Drug Abuse. *Increased Controls over Hallucinogens and Other Dangerous Drugs.* Hearing, 90th Cong., 2d Sess., March 19, 1968. Washington: Government Printing Office, 1968.

———. House and Senate. *Illegal Entry at United States-Mexico Border: Multiagency Efforts Have Not Been Effective in Stemming the Flow of Drugs and People.* Washington: Government Printing Office, 1977.

U.S. Treasury Department. Bureau of Narcotics. *Traffic in Opium and Other Drugs for the Year Ending December 31, 1937.* Washington: Government Printing Office, 1938.

STATE AND FEDERAL LAWS

Title 8 C.F.R. 287.1.
Title 8 U.S. Code 1357a.
Title 21 U.S. Code 841a.
Title 21 U.S. Code 844.
Title 21 U.S. Code 846.
Title 21 U.S. Code 852.
Title 21 U.S. Code 873.

STATE AND FEDERAL COURT CASES

Alexander v. United States, 362 Fed. 2nd (1966).
Boyd v. United States, 116 U.S. 616 (1886).
Brady v. United States, 379 U.S. 752 (1968).
Carroll v. United States, 267 U.S. 134 (1924).
Chimel v. California, 89 S. Ct. Repts. 2034 (1969).
Henderson v. United States, 390 Fed. 2nd (1967).
Landau v. United States, 82 Fed. 2nd (1936).
Lindner v. United States, 268 U.S. 189 (1925).
Mapp v. Ohio, 392 U.S. 643 (1961).
McMann v. Richardson, 397 U.S. 759 (1970).
Parker v. North Carolina, 396 U.S. 759 (1970).
Terry v. Ohio, 392 U.S. 1 (1968).
Thomas v. United States, 372 U.S. 189 (1925).

INDEX

ABOUT THE AUTHOR

Jerald W. Cloyd is a member of the Criminal Justice Department at the State University of New York at Brockport. His articles have appeared in *Social Force*, *Social Problems*, and *Urban Life*.